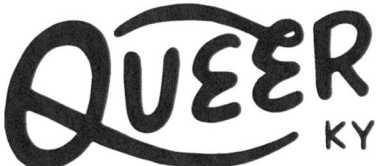

Queer Kentucky is a diverse LGBTQ+ run non-profit based in Louisville, Kentucky working to bolster and enhance Queer culture and health through storytelling, education and action. Through our storytelling approach, we give visibility and celebrate the lives of LGBTQ+ people in the great Bluegrass State. Visibility alone is life-saving. Queer Kentucky actively works with organizations and businesses on their inclusivity efforts that enhance the well-being of their employees.

Dedication
To every queer person struggling and all those that have succumbed to their struggles.
Please know, you aren't alone.

And to the thriving LGBTQ+ people and allies working to enhance the lives of our community.

We see you fighting and we're standing with you.

Copyright © 2023 by Queer Kentucky
All rights reserved.
ISBN: 979-8-9880764-0-7
Queer Kentucky
900 East Main Street
Louisville, KY 40206

MAGAZINE EDITORIAL TEAM

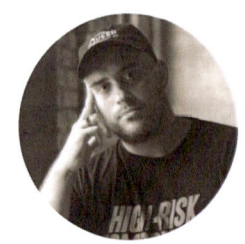

Spencer Jenkins *he/him*
Founder, Executive Director

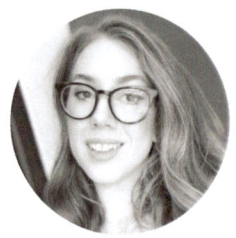

Hallie Decker *she/her*
Associate Editor

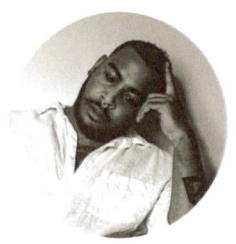

Bearykah Shaw *they/them*
Portrait Photographer

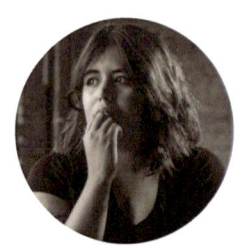

Andy Aliaga-Mendoza *she/her/ella*
Illustrator

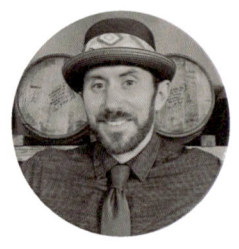

Aaron Thomas *he/him*
Cover Story

INDEX

6	Letter from the Founder
9	Constructs and Potlucks
10	With 11 Anti-LGBTQ+ Bills in KY 2023 Legislative Session, Call This a Battle Cry
15	Gender Euphoria: The Bright Side of Trans Experience
17	Coming Out: A Journey Down to Earth
18	Girls Night In
20	Why Won't My Healthcare Provider Use My Chosen Name?
22	Navigating Healthcare in an Anti-Fat and Anti-Black World
24	Growth from the Shadows
25	Queer Health Clinics: Safe Havens for Queer Patients and Providers
28	We Are Here
30	Ethel Loveless: The Traveling Tangerine Showgirl Creates a Grittier and More Inclusive Nightlife Community
36	Queer Creatives Connect Community Through Nightlife
50	Are Therapists Sufficiently Trained to Help LGBTQ+ Clients?
54	Miniature Self Portraits
56	Access to Trans-Healthcare with Kellee Duke
59	Heart Charmer
60	Gran-Gran
61	Reconcile
62	Microaggressions Matter for Queer Health Justice
65	4 of Hearts
66	HIV Outbreak in Kentucky
70	The Mask
72	Another Sexy Sex Ed Update
76	A Fighting Chance: Queer Youth, Education Equity, and Mental Health
79	Error
80	Body Horror: The Queer and the Macabre
82	Queer, Neurodivergent Entrepreneur Takes a Nonbinary Approach in Helping Autistic Community
86	Ambiguity and Access: Louisville Non-Profit Calls for Legislation to Clarify HIV Self-Testing Regulation in Kentucky

Dear Reader,

A staple of being a suburban 90s baby was going through the drive-through at McDonald's and selecting your toy to go with your Happy Meal. The thought of unlatching the cardboard and being slapped in the face with the smell of hot oil and plastic wrap brings me such nostalgia.

My grandmother, Lois, as I called her by her real name because my family is anything but ordinary, would take me on a Happy Meal run every time I visited her. Whatever I wanted, she'd make sure I'd get it.

All week, I'd watch the commercials on TV showing the fire-striped Hotwheels race cars and beautiful long-haired Barbies in their elegant dresses being placed in each Happy Meal.

"Hot Wheels for the boys and Barbies for the girls!" shouted the voice in the commercials. This was back when verbiage was spewed quickly and aggressively during toy commercials. You know the voice I'm talking about.

But why the gender roles? Did McDonald's have authority on what boys like and what girls like? I didn't want a race car. I had zero interest in them — unless they had a glitter finish. I wanted the Barbie. I wanted to brush her hair, set her up on dates with GI Joes, and make them live happily ever after.

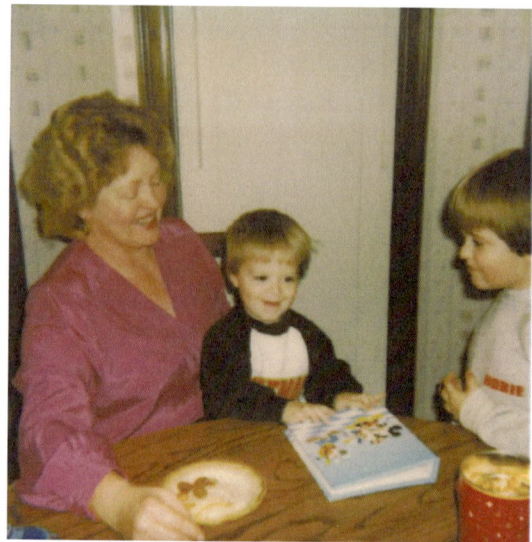

I couldn't tell you why this was the case and honestly, no young child needs to explain why they color outside the lines of gender norms.

Are girls not allowed to drive fast or race cars? Are boys not allowed to feel elegant and beautiful? When we'd roll up to the drive-thru speaker in her 94' Cadillac Sedan de Ville, Lois would order my nugget happy meal and proudly say, "with the Barbie toy, too."

Reflecting on this simple exchange between a loved family member and myself, I realize it was the first time I was affirmed as a queer kid. I was less than 10 years old at this time and I didn't have the language to explain my gratitude for affirmation.

Honestly, this is how easy it is to affirm the life of a queer kid. I cannot even fathom growing up queer right now. Yes, these kids have more peers than me or the generation before me that support and love them, but they also have vile adults pushing them into suicide, self-harm, and addiction.

Please, give a boy a barbie and some glitter. Trust me when I tell you, you'll love seeing him shine.

Love always,
Spencer Jenkins, Founder and Executive Director

www.queerkentucky.com

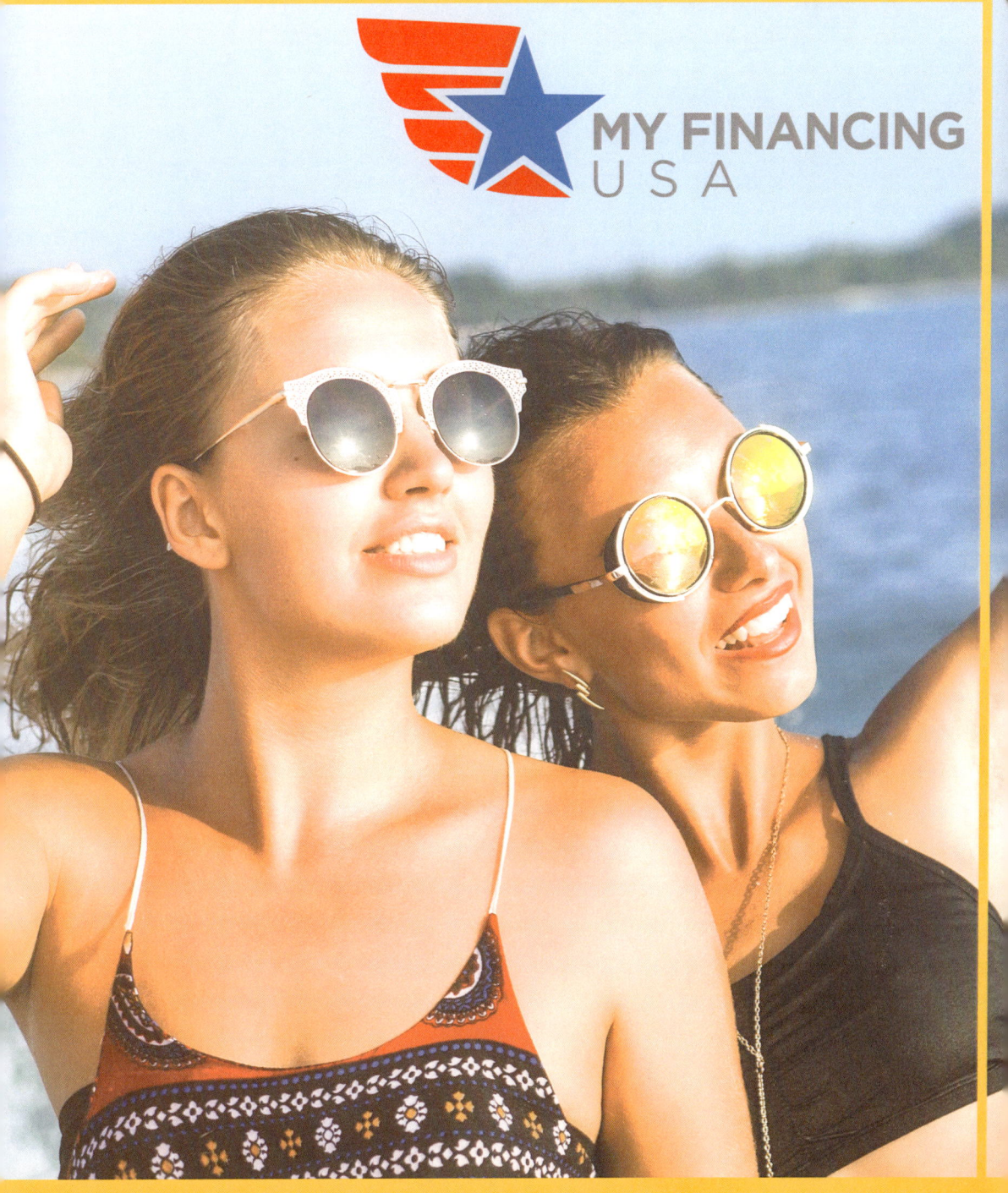

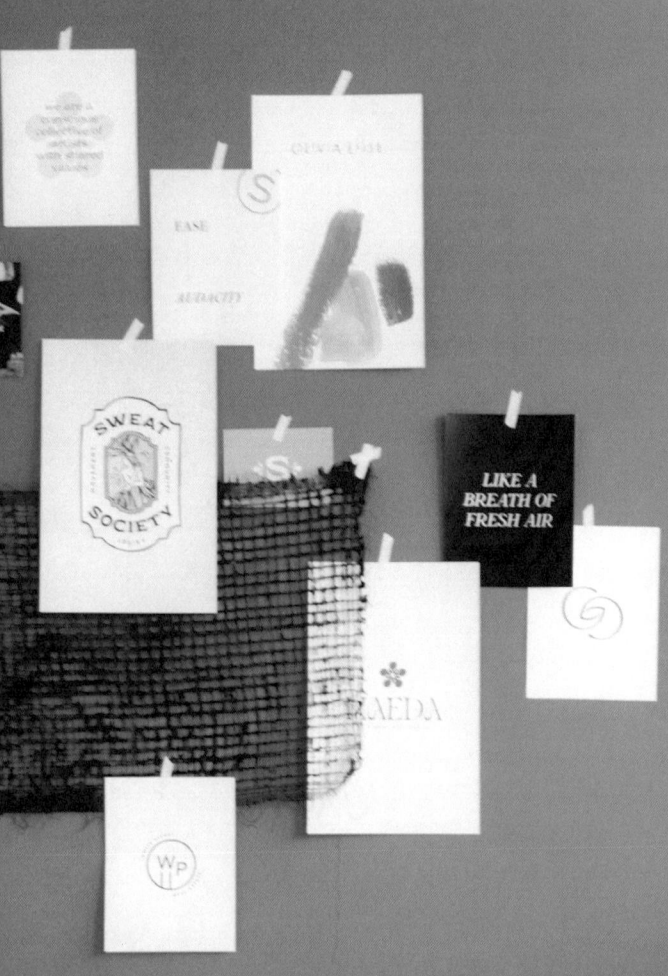

CONSTRUCTS AND POTLUCKS

I grew up Southern Baptist
in the western hills of Kentucky,
where the wind whispers songs
of the beauty in everything.

The bluegrass sits with the wind
long enough to sway with it,
and I sit with the trees long enough
to breathe with them.

Kentucky, where the skies are bigger
and we bring freshly baked
chocolate chip banana bread to the new neighbor.

Home, where the dinner is better
and we bring baskets of homemade casseroles
to the woman who just lost her mom.

I grew up in the western hills of Kentucky,
where the pews and the grocery store aisles whisper
songs of judgment and rejection.

The people cannot sit with themselves
long enough to not be afraid of the unknown,
and I look at them long enough
to let them know that I am still here, anyway.

The land of Kentucky taught me
to be present and take in the moment that I am in.
I am here. Here, I learned to show up for people
right now, because that is all that matters.

Kentucky, where a few people
benefit off of the exploitation and silencing
of many, and many just perpetrate it
because of false moral superiority
and wanting to cash in on whatever social currency
they have to fall back on.

This home of mine has taught me how to be,
and its people have taught me how to be, despite.
Kentucky, oh how you make me grow.

Belle Townsend *she/they*

WITH 11 ANTI-LGBTQ+ BILLS IN KY* 2023 LEGISLATIVE SESSION,

Call This a Battle Cry

Belle Townsend *she/they*

Many people think that LGBTQ+ discrimination is an inherent part of being an out and proud queer person in Kentucky. To some people, it is not a surprise that we are still fighting for LGBTQ+ rights in Kentucky in 2023.

But, I was born and raised in western Kentucky. My neighbors and I made sure each other lived to see another day no matter the differences between us, because our culture taught us that all we have is each other. My culture taught me that we ain't as different as we might seem, and we simple folk will always have more in common than the rich and powerful people who actually call the shots.

This is why I have the hesitant optimism to be surprised that there were 11 anti-LGBTQ+ pieces of legislation making their way through the Kentucky state legislature in 2023.

According to a recent Mason-Dixon Polling and Strategy statewide poll of registered Kentucky voters, 71% opposed medical bans for transgender youth. With 8% of folks undecided, only 21% of Kentucky voters actually support medical bans for transgender youth. Without strategic legislative maneuvers to get the bills voted on quickly and quietly, it is clear that Kentuckians do not want policies that overrule parents' decision to obtain certain healthcare for their teenagers.

Despite specific parts of Kentucky's culture to be welcoming and understanding despite differences, it is undeniable that the intertwined systems of white supremacy, fascism, and capitalism all are at play in continuing to violently erase LGBTQ+ people from existing in this state. As a part of remaining optimistic for LGBTQ+ existence in Kentucky, we must be pessimistic in naming our opposition for what it is. Below are the bills attacking us and our existence in Kentucky, but, make no mistake: the fight ain't over yet.

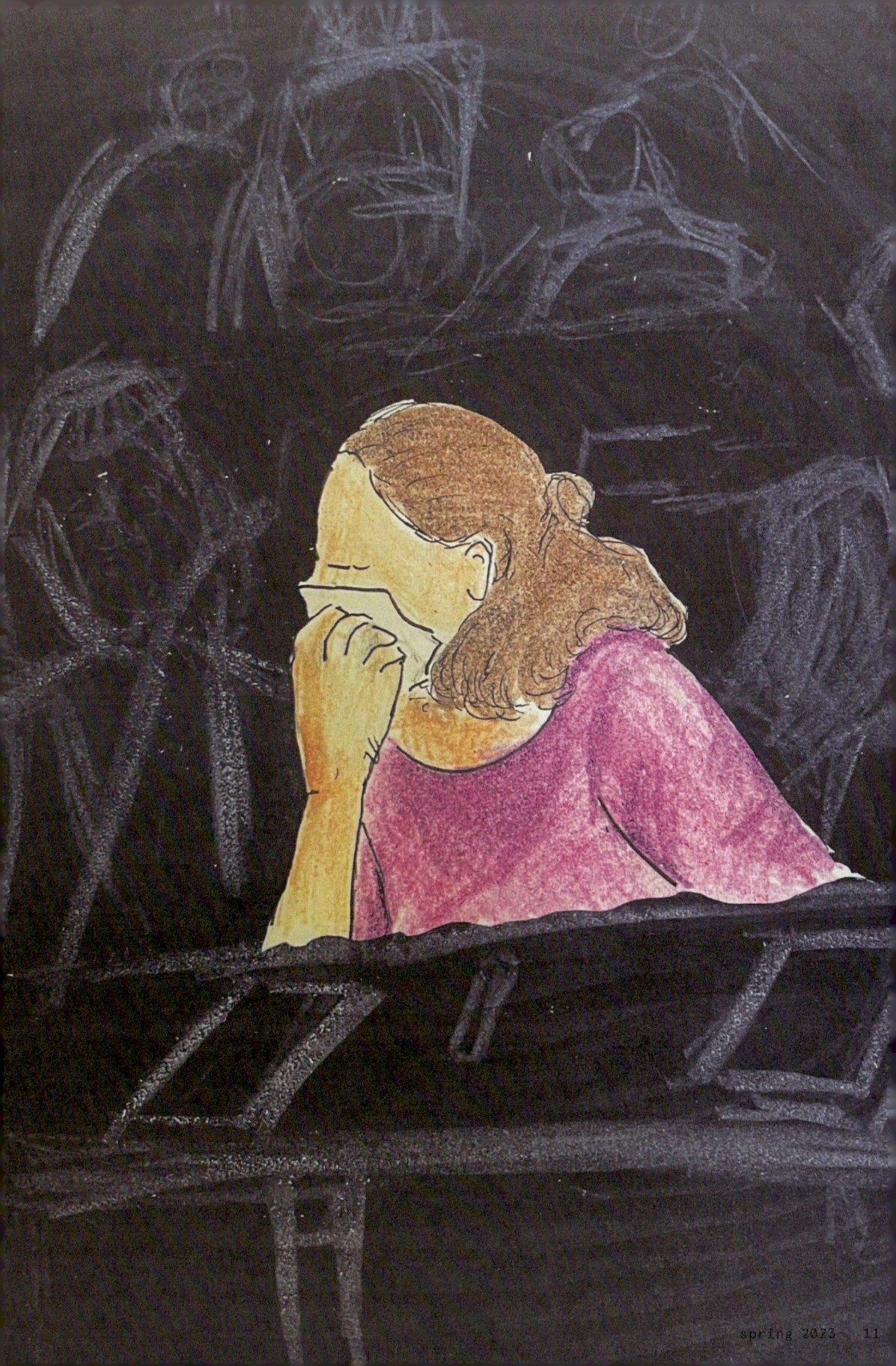

Senate Bill 5

Characterized by critics as a book banning bill, this bill would create a system to allow for parents to allege that materials taught in school are "harmful to minors", effectively creating a complaint resolution policy. The creation of such a system is a part of the conservative movement to oppose Critical Race Theory, a term co-opted by the movement to fearmonger namely white parents into thinking their children are being indoctrinated into the liberal agenda. Such a system creates a greater burden for teachers, detracts from creating systems that are proven to improve ALL student outcomes, and allows for parents to limit their children's worldview: both in the home and in the classroom. It has passed the Senate and House, and now has landed on Governor Andy Beshear's desk.

House Bill 470

This bill "cracks down on gender transition services for any Kentuckian under 18," according to the Lexington Herald-Leader. Further outlined by Herald-Leader's Austin Horn, "The bill defines, 'gender transition services" as "any service provided or performed by a healthcare provider or mental healthcare provider for the purpose of assisting a person with a gender transition." The bill originally passed the House but could not get enough reads to pass before the legislative session ended. Portions of this bill were inserted into SB 150 after it did not make it through the legislature by itself, likely due to such a passionate response from medical professionals, people concerned with government overstep in parental relationships, and folks who understand the necessity of gender affirming care.

House Bill 30

This bill would put heavy restrictions and surveillance on bathrooms, locker rooms, and shower rooms for transgender individuals. It is also stipulated that there are consequences for using facilities designated to the sex not assigned on an unedited birth certificate. This bill did not make it out of comittee.

House Bill 58

This bill would allow for medical providers to decline to perform, participate in, and pay for procedures that violate their "conscience," which is subjective and could be used to discriminate against anyone. This would likely be disproportionately used against Black, brown, and indigenous people of color the most in Kentucky. This bill did not make it to committee.

Senate Bill 120

This bill would prevent minors under 18 from having access to gender transition procedures, as well as limit access to any coverage for gender-affirming care. Access to gender-affirming surgical procedures and hormone regulation therapy is the difference between life or death for many LGBTQ+ youths. This bill did not make it to committee.

Senate Bill 115

This bill has been widely characterized as an anti-drag bill, and a similar one just passed in Tennessee. This bill would regulate both access to and locations of "adult oriented businesses," which would include venues that host drag performances. Effectively, this bill would shut down drag bars, eliminate drag from PRIDE, and discourage bars from hosting drag performances. This bill passed the House, went to Senate, then went back to committee, and never made it back out.

House Bill 173

This bill expands on the conservative education movement advocating for "parental choice" in various areas related to their children's education (similar to SB 150, above). This facade began with discussions surrounding Critical Race Theory, which decentralizes white supremacy in curriculum, and has now moved on to removing any LGBTQ+ stories and media from libraries and classrooms. This bill was withdrawn March 13.

House Bill 177

This bill effectively combines traditional "Don't Say Gay" bills with privacy laws, forcing teachers to out queer children to their parents and banning any discussion of LGBTQ+ topics. This bill never made it out of committee.

Senate Bill 102

This bill would establish a course of action for

a child encountering a person of the opposite biological sex in specific areas, and limit faculty and staff's ability to discuss sexual orientation, preference, and gender expression. It also includes provisions for parents' right for a child to not be exposed to "obscene" matters. It prohibits the "indoctrination" of a student to any "partisan political position," without noting that freedom of gender expression, itself, has been made into a partisan political issue. This bill did not make it out of committee.

House Bill 204

This bill is a sweeping religious freedom bill that would allow people to discriminate against LGBTQ+ folks, Black, brown, and indigenous people of color, and other marginalized groups. This bill could have dismantled all of Kentucky's 24 fairness ordinances, but it did not make it past bouncing around the House committee.

Senate Bill 150

This bill would prohibit school staff and students from being required to use pronouns for gender non-conforming students, as well as increase "parental rights in regard to dictating their child's use of pronouns." This co-opts language from the conservative education movement. Inserted in the last minute, this bill now includes aspects of HB 470, banning gender-affirming medical care for trans youths. Doctors would have to provide a timeline to detransition youth already on puberty blockers or receiving hormone regulation therapy. As well, schools cannot engage in discussions on sexual orientation or gender identity with students of any age. Further, there is a non-specific insertion about "at least" keeping trans kids out of bathrooms tied to their gender identity. This bill served as a Trojan Horse for most of the slate of hate, and it passed the House and Senate. Andy Beshear is anticipated to veto the bill, but after that, the bill would return to the same General Assembly who voted it through. Legislators return March 29, where youth are already organizing a protest to advocate against legislators passing SB 150, from 9:30-11:30 on the steps of the Capitol. Further, if this does pass, the ACLU will likely sue on the grounds of the 14th amendment and equal protection under the law for LGBTQ+ people.

All of these bills are as surprising as they are not. We have lived in Kentucky long enough to understand the nuances of being LGBTQ+ here. But, this outward attack on us will not be as quick and quiet as they want it to b. Politics are ever-changing, with sneaky things happening behind the scenes to get as much of this passed as they can get. It seems right now that SB 5 and SB 150 are the biggest threats, but we will continue updating on social media as changes come.

There are many of us fighting back, and there is still time to fight. As Eastern Kentucky Mutual Aid, @ekymutualaid, said on Twitter,

"We don't know how to stop the fascist legislation that puts our Queer kinfolks and babies in danger. We holler till we're hoarse. We don't know how to shut up… We're here with our hearts in our hands, our hands in yours. We're here with the knowledge of the ones who went before us…It's okay to shut down, to cry, to scream at the sky they've poisoned over our heads. We know our pain ain't removed from righteous anger. We're all we've got y'all.

Get mad. Get together. We love you."

CHEAT SHEET	SB5	HB470	SB150	HB30	HB58
SB120	SB115	HB173	HB177	SB102	HB204

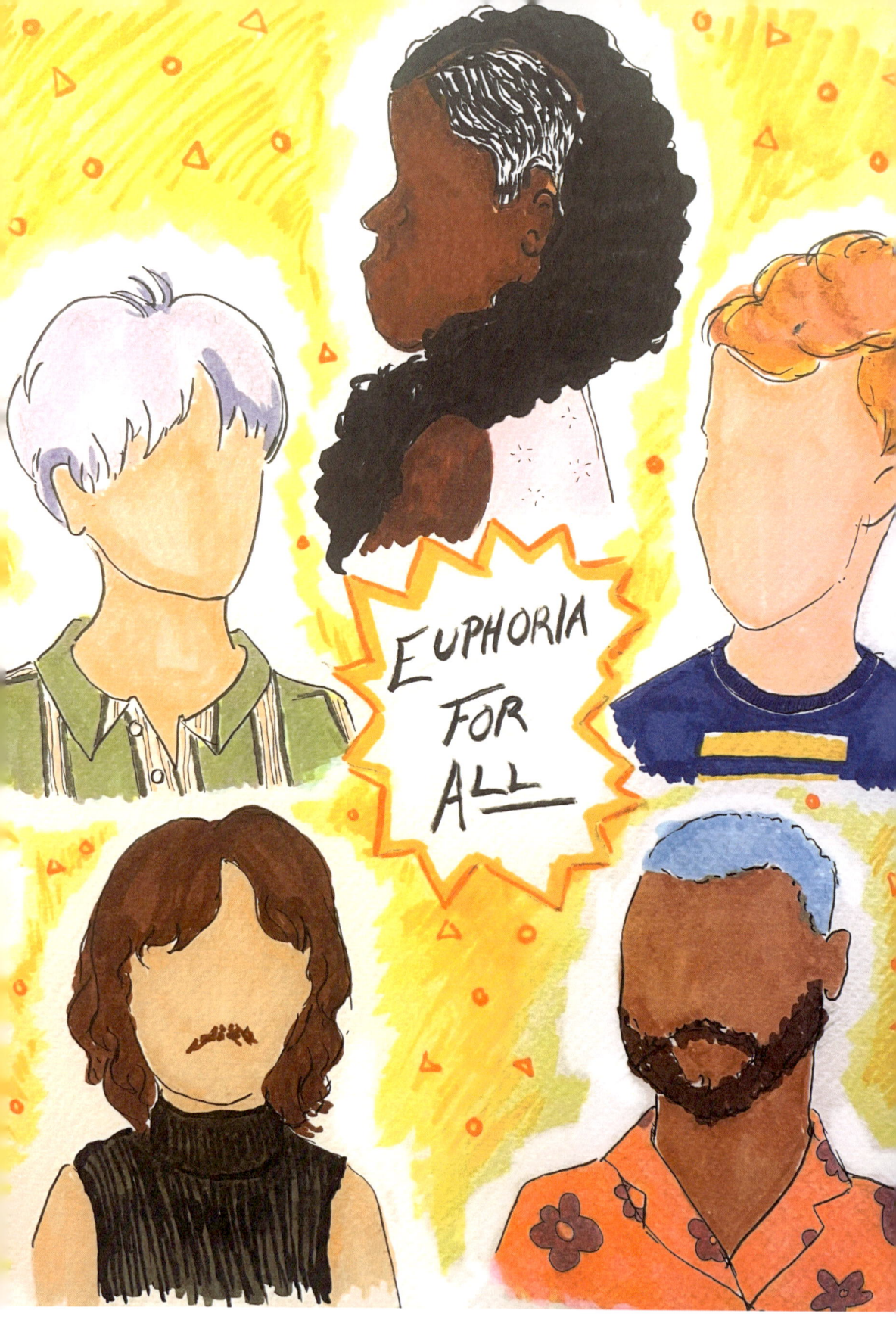

Gender Euphoria: The Bright Side of Trans Experience

Adrian Silbernagel he/him

Some of us figure out we're trans the moment we're first introduced to the gender binary ("mama or dada," "brother or sister," "boy or girl.") Others perform countless variations of our assigned gender before realizing that all of them somehow feel equally wrong.

Some of us wake up one day knowing, and never look back. Others spend years chipping away at layer after layer of fear, shame, guilt, denial, social and/or familial expectations, before arriving at our "true gender," or a self-expression that feels right to us. For some, it just takes a simple thought experiment: "If I could go back in time and change my assigned gender, would I?" Or: "If no one else had an opinion, how would I identify?" And for others it takes experimenting with clothing, presentation, pronouns, names, etc. before they figure out what feels right.

In the US, the aspect of trans experience that doctors and psychologists and the media fixate on is dysphoria: the experience of discomfort, dissatisfaction, or distress over the wrongness or incongruity between the trans person's internal and external reality, between their sex and gender, body and mind, presentation and inner sense of self.

This fact is at once cause and symptom of the medicalization and pathologization of trans people in the US. I say "in the US" because, contrary to popular opinion, trans people have existed and have been accepted as valid in many other parts of the world throughout human history. But in the US, trans-ness is still seen as synonymous with illness, as pathology; and the textbook narrative, which informs media portrayals of trans people, is defined by negative feelings and experiences.

Every trans person is unique. For me, gender expression was the gateway to understanding gender identity, and it took moving several states away from my family before I felt comfortable taking steps toward a gender expression that felt like home.

Within just a couple of weeks of moving to Lubbock, Texas for grad school, I cut my hair. A week later, I cut it again, this time shorter, and more squarely. At the local Goodwill, I nonchalantly browsed the perimeter of the men's clothing section, avoiding any and all eye contact, until the coast was clear and I could make a bee-

Artwork by Andy Mendoza she/her/ella

> **GENDER EUPHORIA:**
>
> the feeling of satisfaction, joy, or intoxication, with the congruence, or rightness, between one's internal and external reality (sex and gender, internal experience and outside expression, etc.)

line for it. I grabbed heaps of musty button down shirts, men's jeans and shorts, sad-looking shoes—really anything that looked remotely close to my size would do—and then booked it to the gender-neutral dressing room.

In the dressing room, I watched myself transform into the handsome devil I secretly believed I could be. I stood in awe of my new, more definitively masculine figure and aesthetic, and experienced a high I'd never felt before. Trans folks refer to this high as "gender euphoria"—the feeling of satisfaction, joy, or intoxication, with the congruence, or rightness, between one's internal and external reality (sex and gender, internal experience and outside expression, etc.).

I would go on to experience this high, this gender euphoria, countless more times over the next ten years. When I bought my first cologne. When I put on my first binder, pulled my t-shirt back on over it, then looked in the mirror. When I looked down after top surgery, and saw my completely flat chest for the first time ever. When someone called me "sir" for the first time. Or the first time a barista wrote my chosen name on my iced coffee. I could go on.

I was experiencing gender euphoria long before I knew that I was trans—and long before I had language for my experience. For a long time, I really didn't know what to make of it (literally, the first time a stranger "sir'd" me on accident, I was ecstatic and then confused by my own ecstasy.) But a pattern emerged, a pattern which would eventually lead me to an understanding of my gender.

But it's not just me. Gender euphoria is an essential part of many trans people's experience and journey of self-discovery. Despite its prevalence, euphoria is not something that most cis people (or non-trans people) would think to associate with trans experience.

In reality, however, gender euphoria is just as essential (if not more so) to many trans folks' narratives as dysphoria is. It's time cis people, especially those who treat trans people, or who write us into their plot lines, became aware of this.

COMING OUT:
A JOURNEY DOWN
TO EARTH

Josiah Rogers
they/them

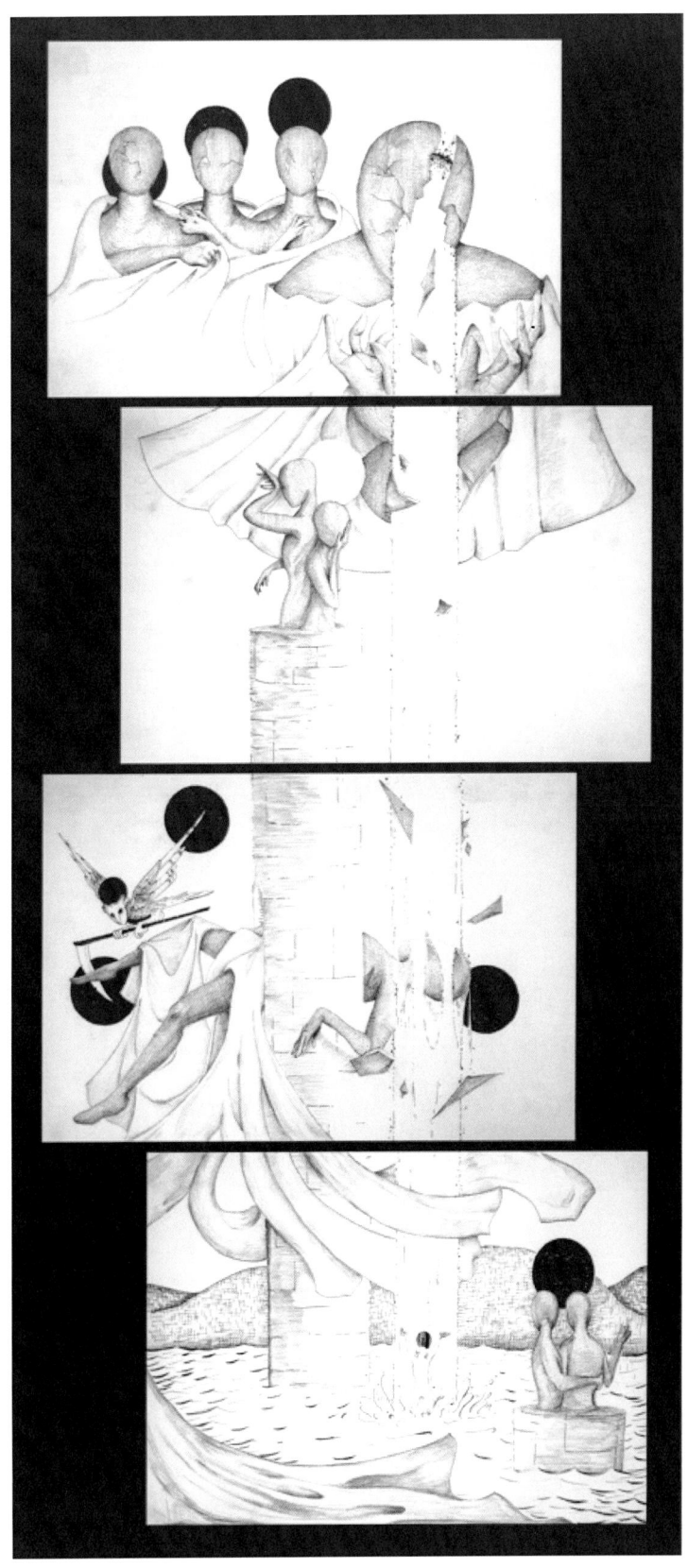

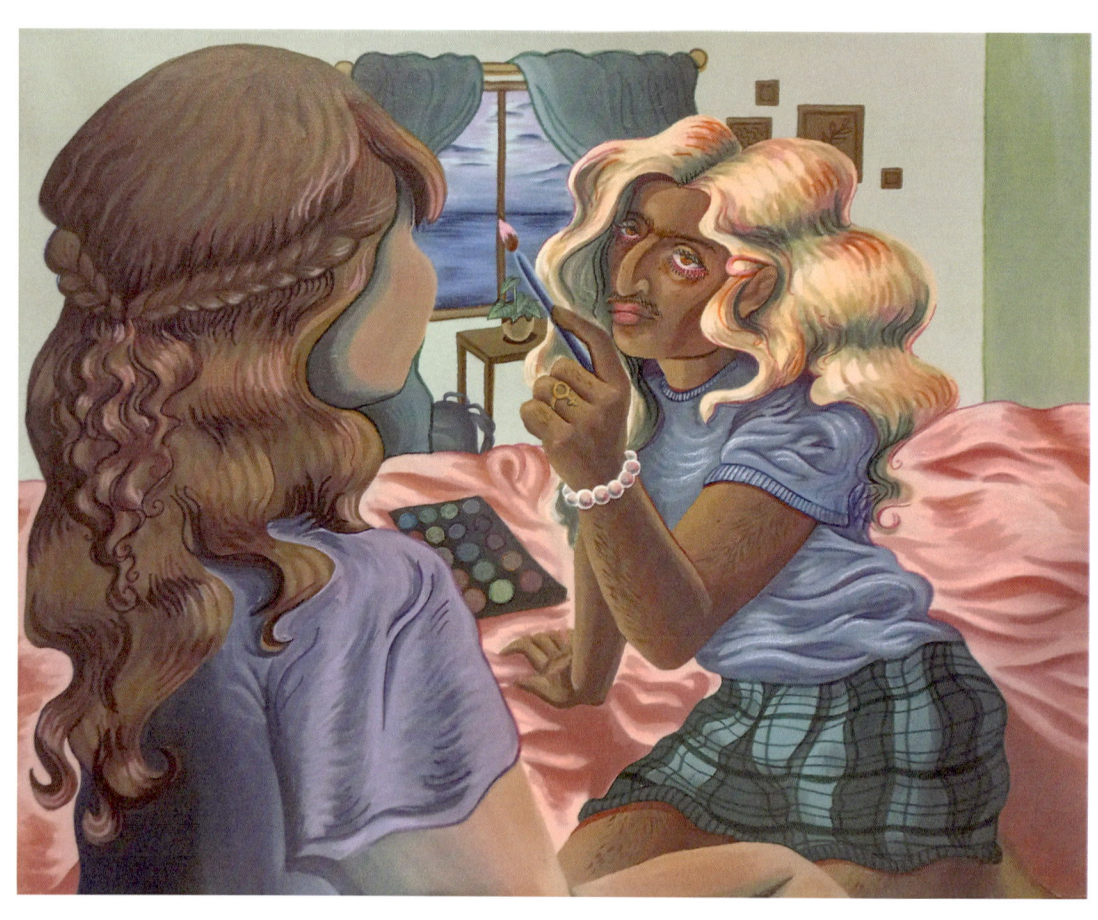

GIRLS NIGHT IN
Simone Jackson *he/she/they*

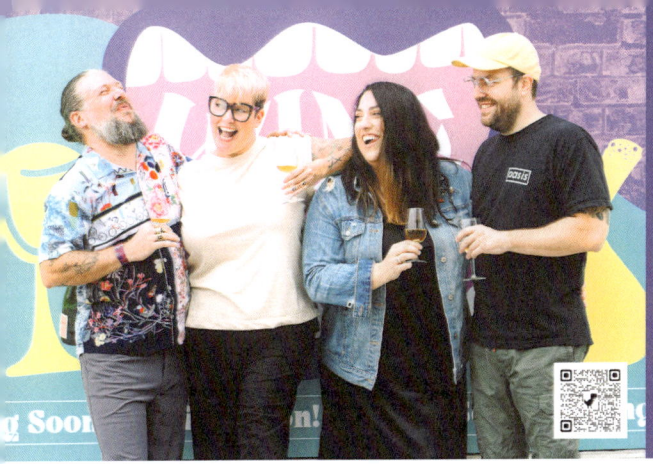
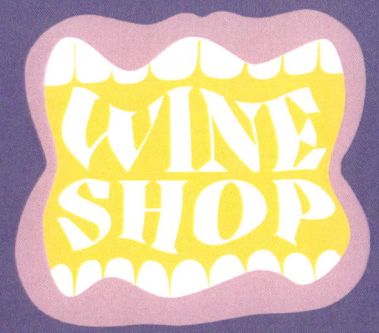

WINE BAR & SPECIALITY BOUTIQUE
WWW.WINESHOPNEWALBANY.COM

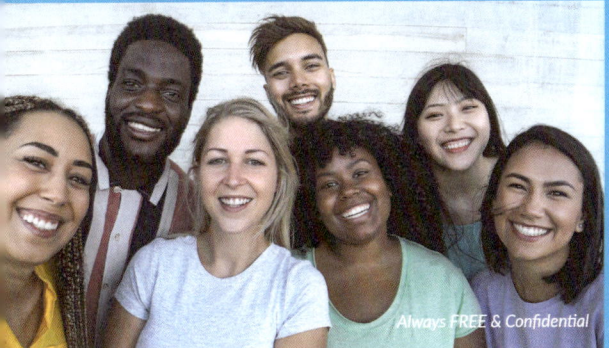

in 7 people living with HIV don't know they are infected.

So, get tested today.

Offering a Continuum of Services to End HIV including: HIV testing, STI testing, connectivity to health insurance and care, and PrEP navigation.

Always FREE & Confidential

AVOL KENTUCKY INC.

1824 Hill Rise Drive, Suite 100
Lexington KY 40504

(859) 225-3000   www.avolky.org

11

anti-LGBTQ+ pieces of legislation are making their way through the Kentucky state legislature in 2023.

Learn how to help at
www.fairness.org

Why Won't My Healthcare Provider Use My Chosen Name?

April McGregor-Bennett, MSN, RN she/her

Why won't my doctor's office respect my chosen name or pronouns? While many healthcare practitioners are striving to be more inclusive in their forms and documentation, many patients still run into problems with being misgendered or dead-named during healthcare appointments. This can be a very triggering experience for many patients, but there is often more behind this issue than a lack of awareness or respect.

Our current healthcare system relies on information known as 'patient identifiers' which allows everyone from the receptionist to the physician or nurse practitioner to be sure that they are speaking to the correct person. This protects patients in many ways, such as from having their private medical information given out incorrectly, or making sure that the nurse is administering medication to the correct person. The two most commonly used patient identifiers are name and date of birth, but can include other things such as patient photos.

So why can't they use my chosen name instead of my legal name? In many cases, this is due to insurance and billing issues. Many facilities use electronic health records, or EHR systems, which allow for easier documentation and billing. However, these systems are usually not designed to allow for alternative names, and must match the name on a patient's insurance card and photo ID. In order for the office to bill your insurance, they have to show that they provided treatment to the person covered by the insurance, which they do by providing information contained in the EHR.

Alright, so they have to have my legal name and sex on file, but why can't they respect my chosen name and pronouns during my appointments? That part is a bit more tricky, but also in many ways comes back to the EHR system. Even if the system used allows for a different name or pronouns to be listed, this information is usually buried somewhere in the system, and is not what is displayed on the screen when the nurse or provider is checking your record during your appointment. A provider who is a strong ally may already be aware of this shortcoming in their system and have created workarounds to ensure that they are using the correct name and pronouns, especially if they see that patient regularly. However, if you only see your provider a few times each year, they are unlikely to personally remember you well enough to realize that they are dead-naming or misgendering you.

What can I do about this? This is where being your own advocate comes in. When you make your appointment, remind the receptionist of your correct name and pronouns. You may also need to remind them when you check in for the appointment. Hopefully, the receptionist will pass this along before you are called back to the exam room, but if not, you may have to remind the nurse as well. A good nurse will make sure to let the practitioner know before they come in. While your healthcare provider may not have any control over the EHR system, as these systems can cost thousands of dollars, they may be open to hearing ideas of other ways they can make their practice more inclusive.

Artwork by Andy Mendoza she/her/ella

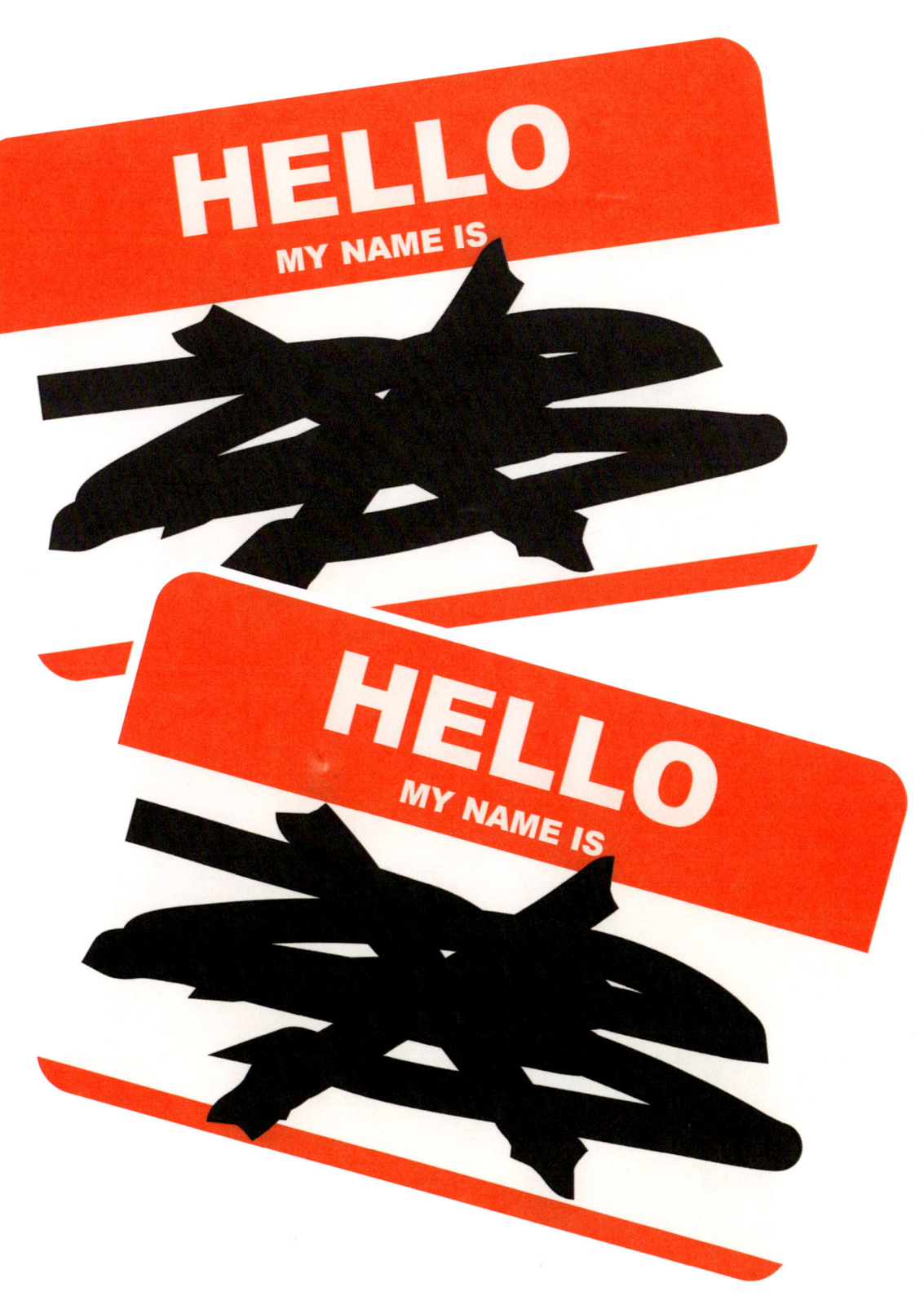

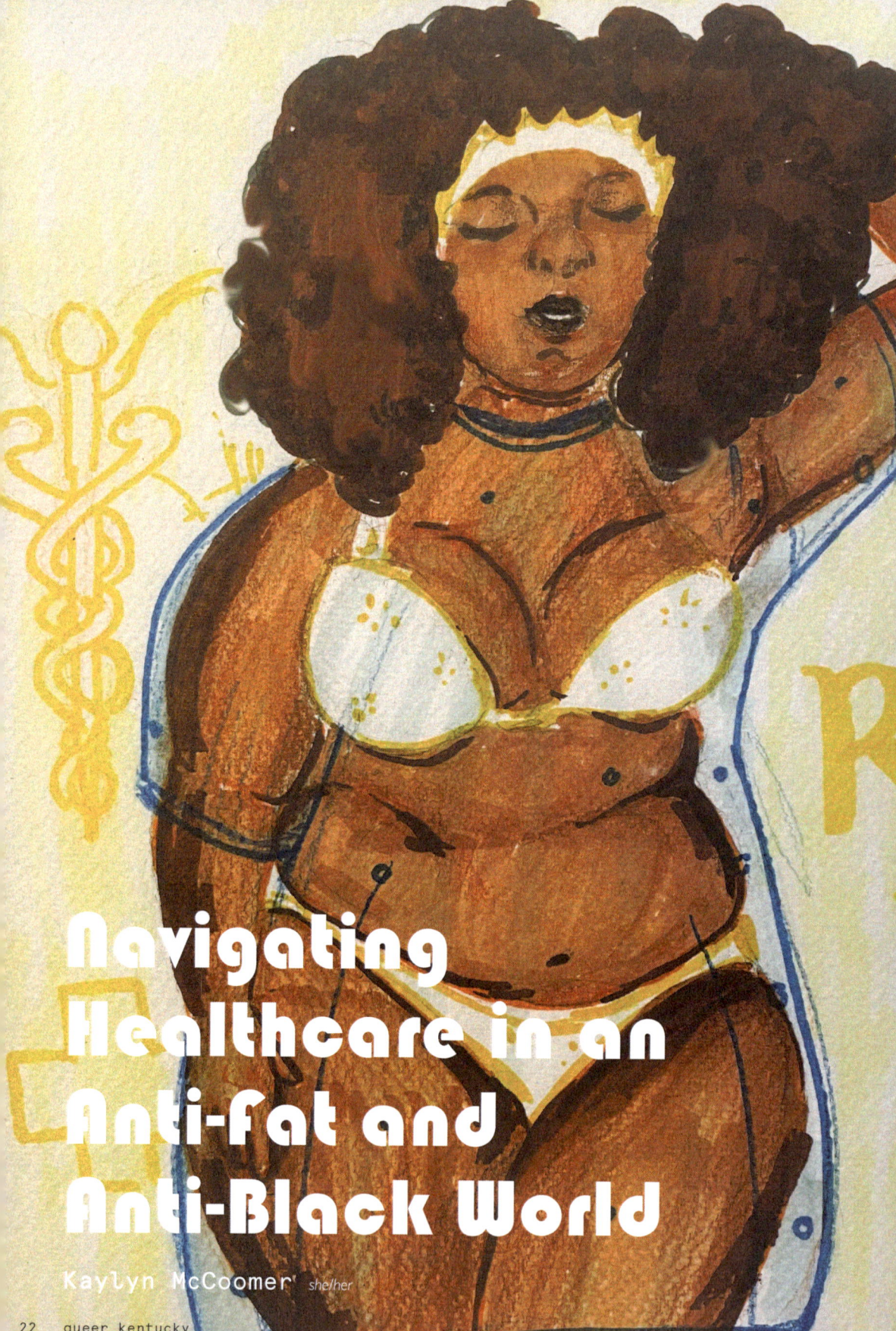

Navigating Healthcare in an Anti-Fat and Anti-Black World

Kaylyn McCoomer *she/her*

At the time, I couldn't name the feeling. How can a child, no older than ten-years-old, articulate the unique discomfort of a cold, sterile exam room while adults discuss her weight? Already so used to bottling up my feelings, I sat there trying to choke back tears, the tingle in the back of my throat intensifying with every word that made me fold into myself. High cholesterol. Diet. Lose weight. By the end of the appointment, my pediatrician became another person who made me ashamed of my weight. Another reason to cower and fold into myself. Another lived experience to build onto my impenetrable walls of safety. Those words, dripped in concern and laced with disdain, hurt me.

I walked out of the office with my head hung low in shame and my own weight on my shoulders, almost like the innocence of childhood was taken from me. I had to grow up with a big, fat monster hovering over me, reminding me that I'm not like others. I'm damaged and should be ashamed for the way my body looks. Negative body image has entered the chat, right at the start of my adolescence and the "Childhood Obesity Epidemic."

On October 26, 1999, the CDC (Centers of Disease Control and Prevention) posted a press release to name and address the problem that needed to be eradicated by any means. In the press release, then CDC director, Jeffery P. Koplan, expressed grave concern about overweight and physically inactive Americans, stating "obesity is an epidemic and should be taken as seriously as any infectious disease epidemic" (CDC, 1999). Suddenly, fat bodies are classified as diseased and inherently bad, a moral failing of the people living in those bodies. Additionally, this classification created a more acute fear of "catching" fatness, and a desperation to police and get rid of fatness, and opened an even larger market for the weight loss industry.

Although the extremities taken to treat obesity puts the lives of fat people at risk, Cardel and Taveras (2020) suggests a cost-benefit analysis of treatment and potential risks of those treatments. They specifically name disordered eating as a risk, and despite the fact that eating disorders "carry one of the highest mortality risks of any psychiatric disorder," they continue to suggest that "obesity treatment programs must consider the balance between the harms of excess weight and those that may occur from weight management." When weight is used as a measure of health, losing weight is always the "cure". Scientific conclusions like those that prioritize weight loss over lives, aid in the dehumanization of fat people, and lead to medical professionals disregarding symptoms and misdiagnoses for fat people.

Within minutes of my first appointment with a new primary care physician, I was asked if I want to lose weight because I'm a great candidate for weight loss surgery. After reluctantly saying yes (because that's what I should want, right?), he gave a list of documentaries to watch. One of those being Fat, Sick, and Nearly Dead, a documentary about a man drinking only fruit and vegetable juice for 60 days. A healthcare professional suggested a documentary that showed disordered eating habits. After a few more visits I stopped going, and that experience aided in my reluctance to seek treatment, which significantly informs my slight case of hypochondria. That anxiety I experience about any health symptoms is one of the main causes of my panic attacks. Knowing that my Blackness and fatness will cause health professionals to not take my symptoms seriously and make me feel embarrassed about my weight, I hesitated on seeking help until I start thinking about my ignored symptoms possibly leading to my death.

I now feel comfortable with most of my physicians; that feeling of shame is not so haunting, and I am more equipped with the knowledge and more confident in advocating for myself. Not everyone has those tools, nor should they be expected to fight systemic health inequities. The onus should be on health professionals, teaching more compassionate care, and educating them on the ways systemic discrimination impacts the healthcare marginalized communities receive.

Artwork by Andy Mendoza she/her/ella

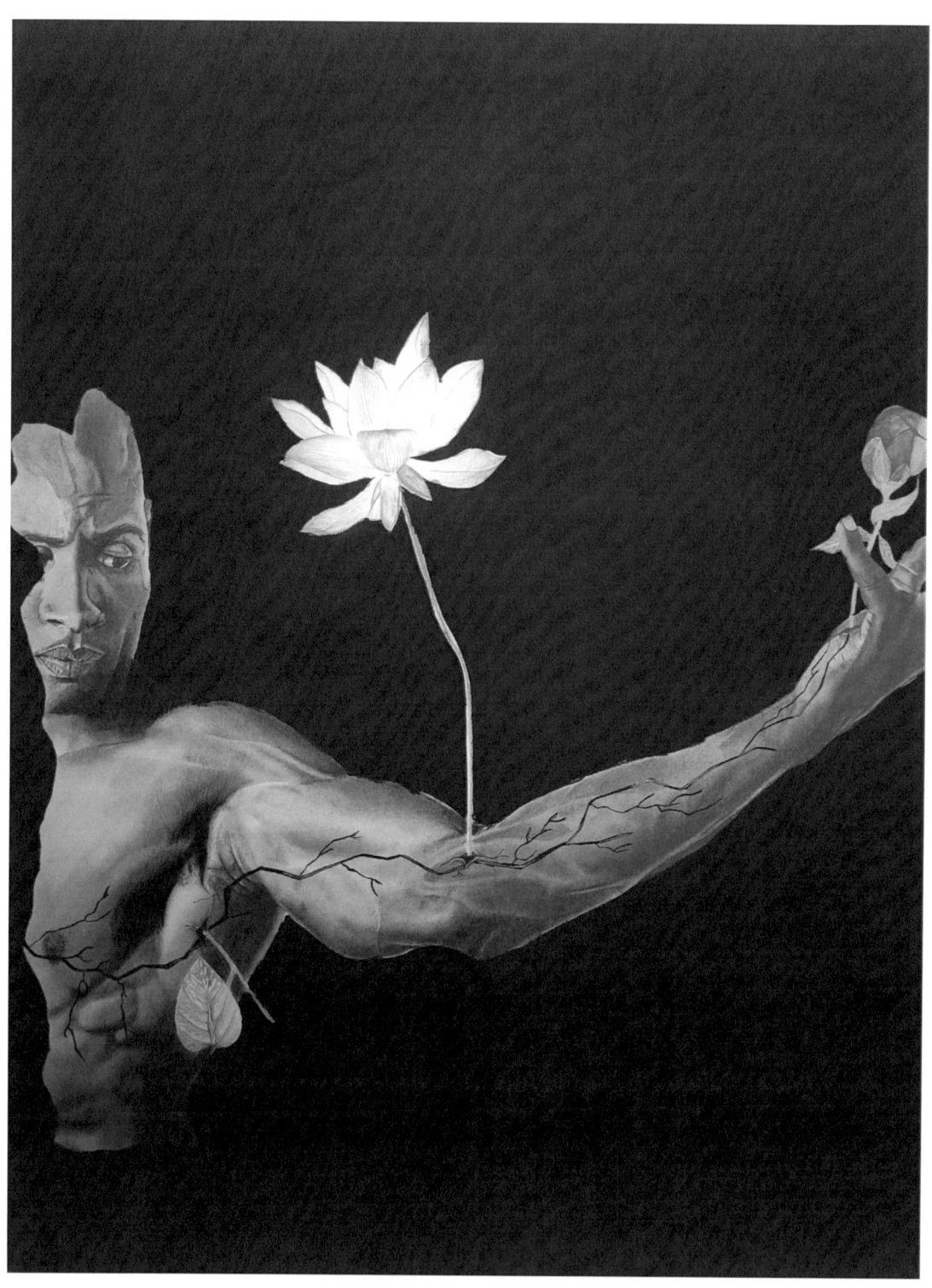

GROWTH FROM THE SHADOWS
Erica Chinise *she/her*

Queer Health Clinics:
Safe Havens for Queer Patients and Providers

Bridget Pitcock *they/she*

Queer health clinics aren't just a safe haven for patients trying to navigate a system that wasn't made for them. They're also a haven for queer healthcare providers. Our healthcare system was built by and for straight, white, cisgender men. Medical research and training are often based on them, too.

No matter how hard I've tried to fit into this world, I've always felt I'm on the outside looking in. Anytime I've changed jobs, the excitement has been overshadowed by the anxiety and dread of having to continuously "come out" to my colleagues. I've watched my cis-hetero friends make long-lasting friendships, whereas I've always found it hard to make those close connections. Often, I have felt that people don't get me – at least not without a lot of extra work on my part. I can make small talk with the best of them. I have even been told I am a likable person! But deeper connections have always been harder.

I'm a queer non-binary femme. Cue me accepting a job as a Nurse Practitioner (NP) in a queer clinic in New York City. I relocated from my home state of Kentucky to take my dream job – to serve LGBTQIA+ people in healthcare. I (temporarily) left my wife and our dogs behind at home, and for 12 months I trained as a primary care provider in one of the largest and longest-running LGBTQIA+ health clinics in New York City.

I've been a nurse for 13 years and an NP for 2.5 years. Even after nearly two decades in the medical field, this job in NYC was the first time I felt like I fit into the world of healthcare. I've always known I was meant to work in this field, but I'd never felt like I belonged. Before I started the job, I realized that the anxiety regarding my sexual orientation and gender identity wasn't there. I wouldn't have to come out to my coworkers. I wouldn't need to explain myself, my life, or the way I present. Instead, I would be able to focus on the position itself, the knowledge I was going to gain, and most importantly, how I could care for my patients. When I realized this, I was astounded. Wow! This is what it should feel like to start a new job!

Walking into the clinic, I realized I didn't have to hide any part of me. I'd been used to predominately straight, white colleagues. Now my colleagues were Black, queer, trans, Latinx, nonbinary, Muslim, and Asian. My supervisor was a transgender NP. My mentor was an out, queer femme physician who'd been taking care of our community since the beginning of the HIV/AIDS epidemic.

Artwork by Andy Mendoza she/her/ella

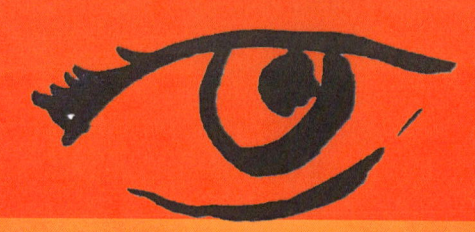
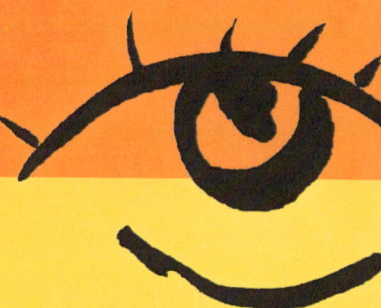
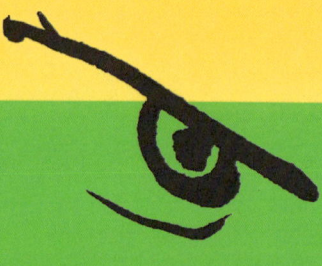
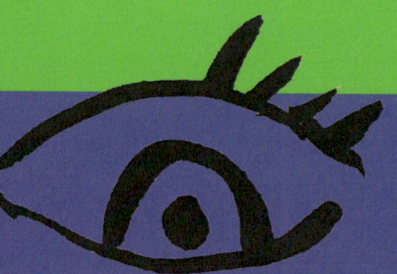
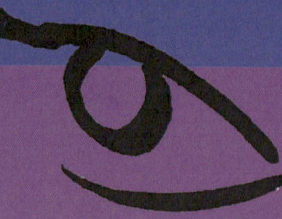

My heart soared. Finally seeing people like me, seeing the possibilities, and having access to specialized expertise and knowledge (e.g. hormone therapy, HIV care, gender-affirming practices) was such a welcome change. This information should be shared in every primary care setting, but sadly it's not.

People often ask me what it was like to move from Kentucky to NYC. Wasn't it a culture shock? My answer is always no. It was nothing short of amazing. I felt like my true self for the first time. I felt fully seen as a healthcare provider.

Coming back to Kentucky was a culture shock. Equipped with all this new knowledge, I headed back home. Upon starting a new job in Kentucky, I was quickly reminded how lucky I had been in NYC. For example, after meeting a colleague at my new job and saying I was married, the next question was, "What does your husband do?" My heart sank. It might seem like a small thing, but folks in the LGBTQIA+ community know it's not. Questions like this, while well-intentioned, make it difficult to be our true selves. I was back to explaining, correcting, and coming out. I realized the unique safe haven my clinic in NYC truly was. It wasn't just an affirming space for our patients – it was an affirming and needed space for me and for queer healthcare providers too.

I wanted to be back in a safe place, and now I am – this time as a remote medical provider, treating LGBTQIA+ patients in NY. I truly believe my skillset can benefit Louisville and the Kentuckiana region. That's why I started "BP the Queer NP" – an organization dedicated to providing education and training to medical providers on LGBTQIA+ terminology, culture, gender-affirming practices, hormone therapy, and HIV care in Kentuckiana.

Louisville needs a queer clinic. It has for years. We need a clinic that serves all queer, trans, and gender-diverse patients – not just those who can afford it or who have insurance. There are incredible affirming providers in Louisville, but having dedicated spaces created by and for us is life-changing – for our patients, our community as a whole, and for ourselves.

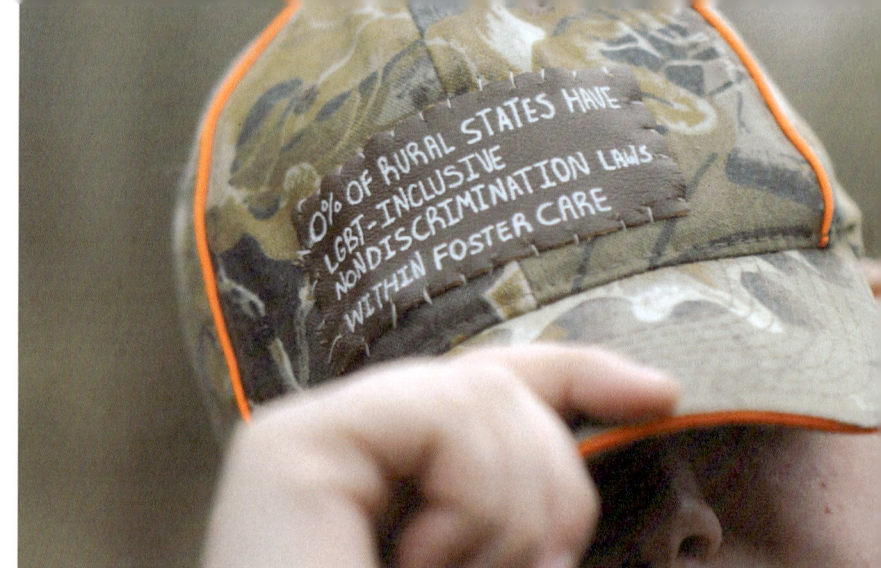

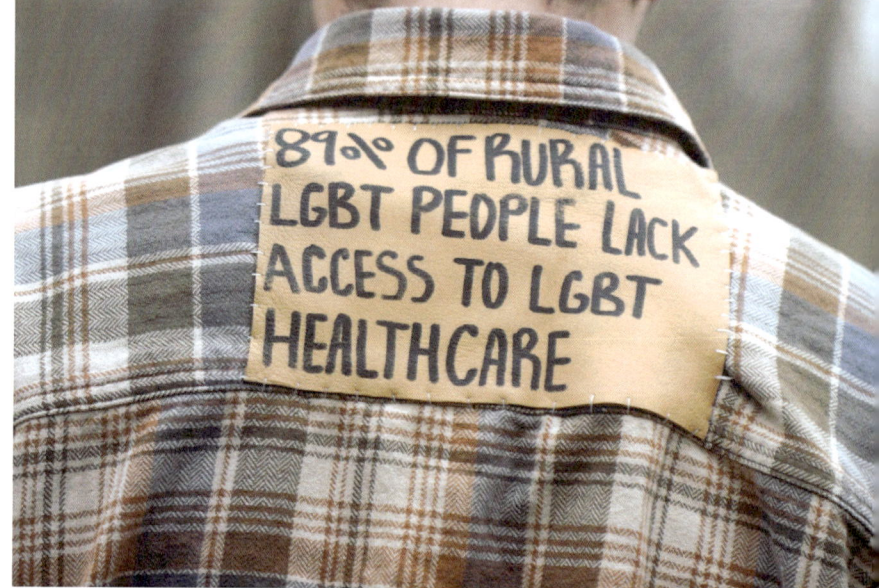

WE ARE
HERE

Alex
Selby
he/him

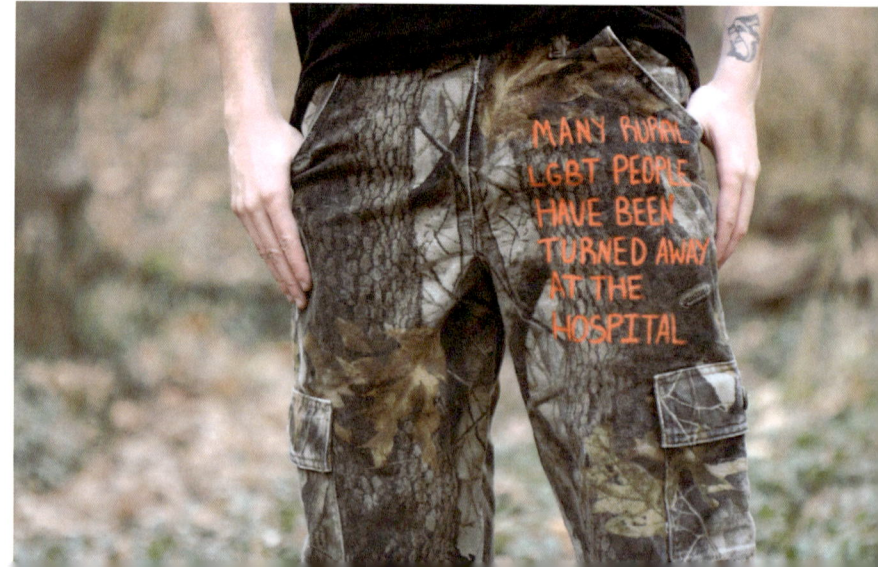

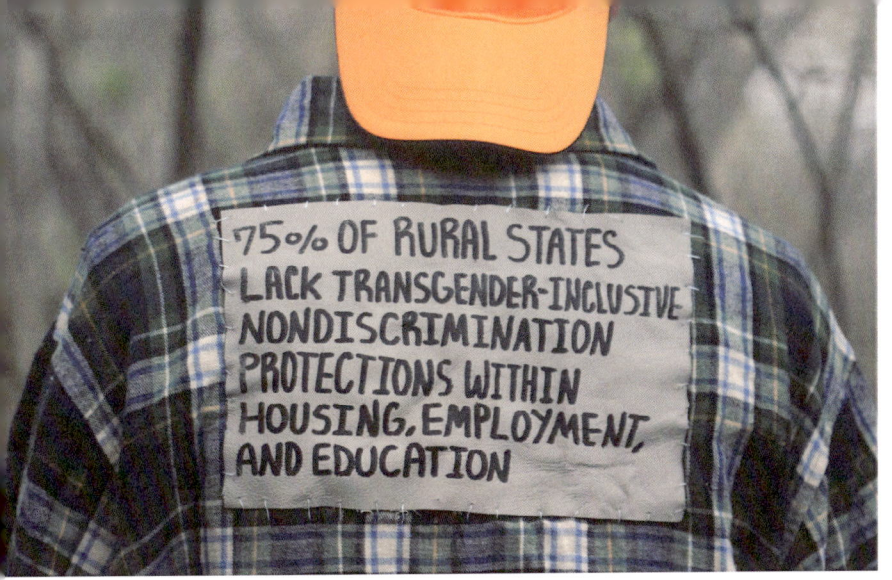

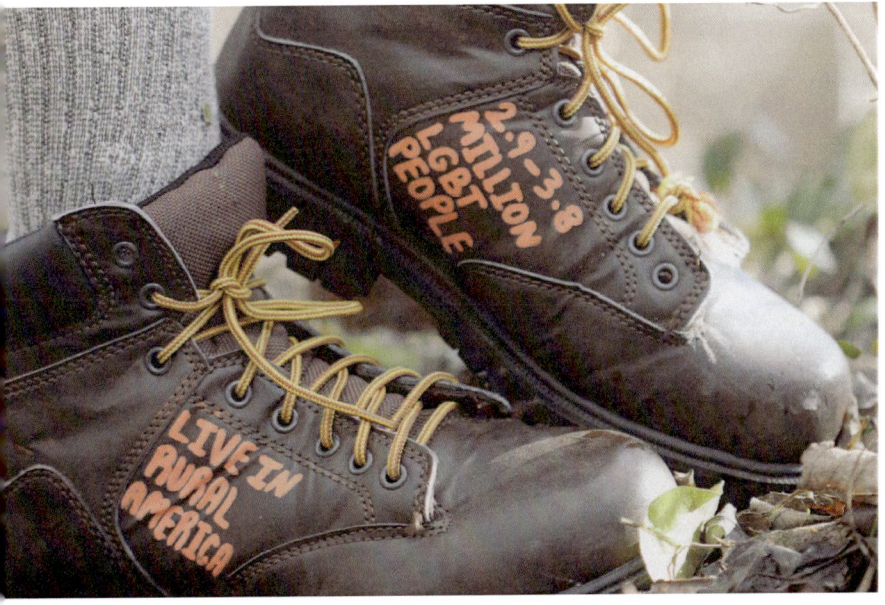

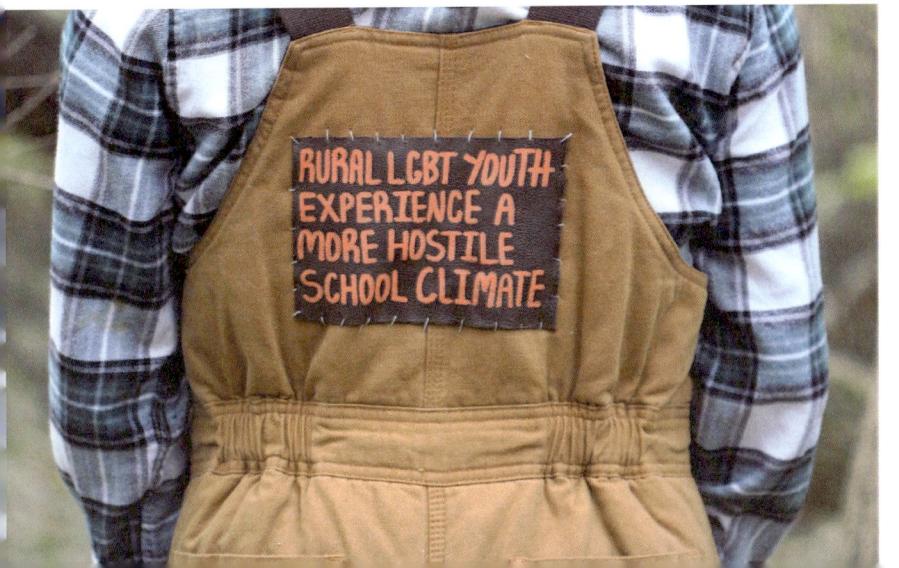

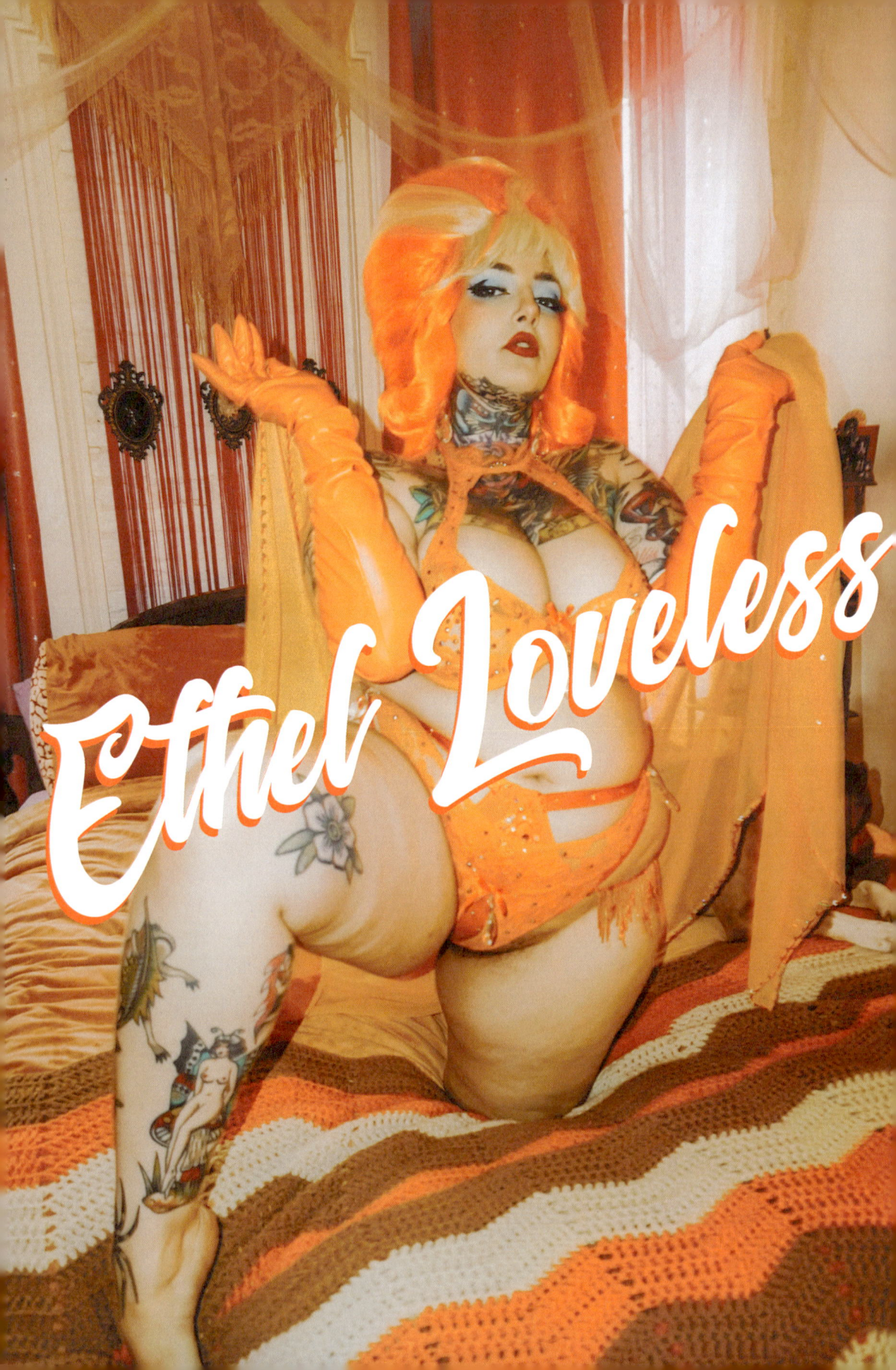

THE TRAVELING TANGERINE SHOWGIRL CREATES A GRITTIER AND MORE INCLUSIVE NIGHTLIFE COMMUNITY

Spencer Jenkins *he/him*

Throughout my career as a professional queer journalist, I have met a circus of people from every corner of the world. From famous Ru girls to trail-blazing activists and politicians; from Queer Eye's Carson Kressley to comedy darlings Matteo Lane and Fortune Feimster; my career has provided me endless opportunities to meet and network with the gayest of gay. However, one will always stand out to me more than the rest because of their vulgar tongue, show-stopping charisma and undying love for the queer community.

Ethel Loveless, who has by all means earned "Mother!" status amongst Kentucky queers, is one of the sole reasons Queer Kentucky exists.

Queer Kentucky was in its infancy and Loveless was twirling tassels on her titties every Tuesday at the Limbo Lounge in downtown Louisville. During that time, "Titty Tiki Tuesday" was the antithesis of a mainstream drag show. Performances were raw, amateur, and sometimes sloppy. Part of the shtick was that performers wouldn't know which song would be played for their performance. I'll never forget the oh-so-blasphemous drag king dressed as a half-naked Jesus or the night I was introduced to Burlesque and Boylesque. As Andy Warhol was to Max's Kansas City or Edie Sedgewick was to his factory, Loveless was to Titty Tiki Tuesday.

Limbo Lounge, owned by Olivia Griffin, was a Tiki-themed bar that the queers claimed rather quickly. Griffin moved to Kentucky from San Francisco in 2014 and realized Louisville had no tiki bar. She had spent her 20s experiencing the wonders of classic Bay Area tiki bars like Smuggler's Cove, Forbidden Island, and Trader Sam's, so she knew that Kentucky needed something of the like. The bar became a thriving hub for Louisville's queer scene, and Titty Tiki Tuesday was a mainstay for the community. However, the bar closed at the end of 2022.

Every Tuesday seemed to embody a wild outtake from John Waters' "Pink Flamingos" - and if you were around Limbo during this time, I know you know what I'm talking about. The bathrooms saw their fair share of sexy rendezvous and powder sniffing. If you were lucky, you'd have a chance to sneak off with one of the sailors hat-wearing bartenders or at least get a little smooch from them across the bar. We played with gender and we played with each other. A hedonistic queer haven? Maybe.

The soundtrack to the Waters' movie never created about Kentucky fried queers in a dark dive was curated by two of my most precious queer comrades, DJ Spring Break (Duncan Cherry) and DJ Syimone.

And yes, the traveling tangerine queen, Ethel Loveless, was our naughty emcee.

Photos by Bearykah Shaw   they/them

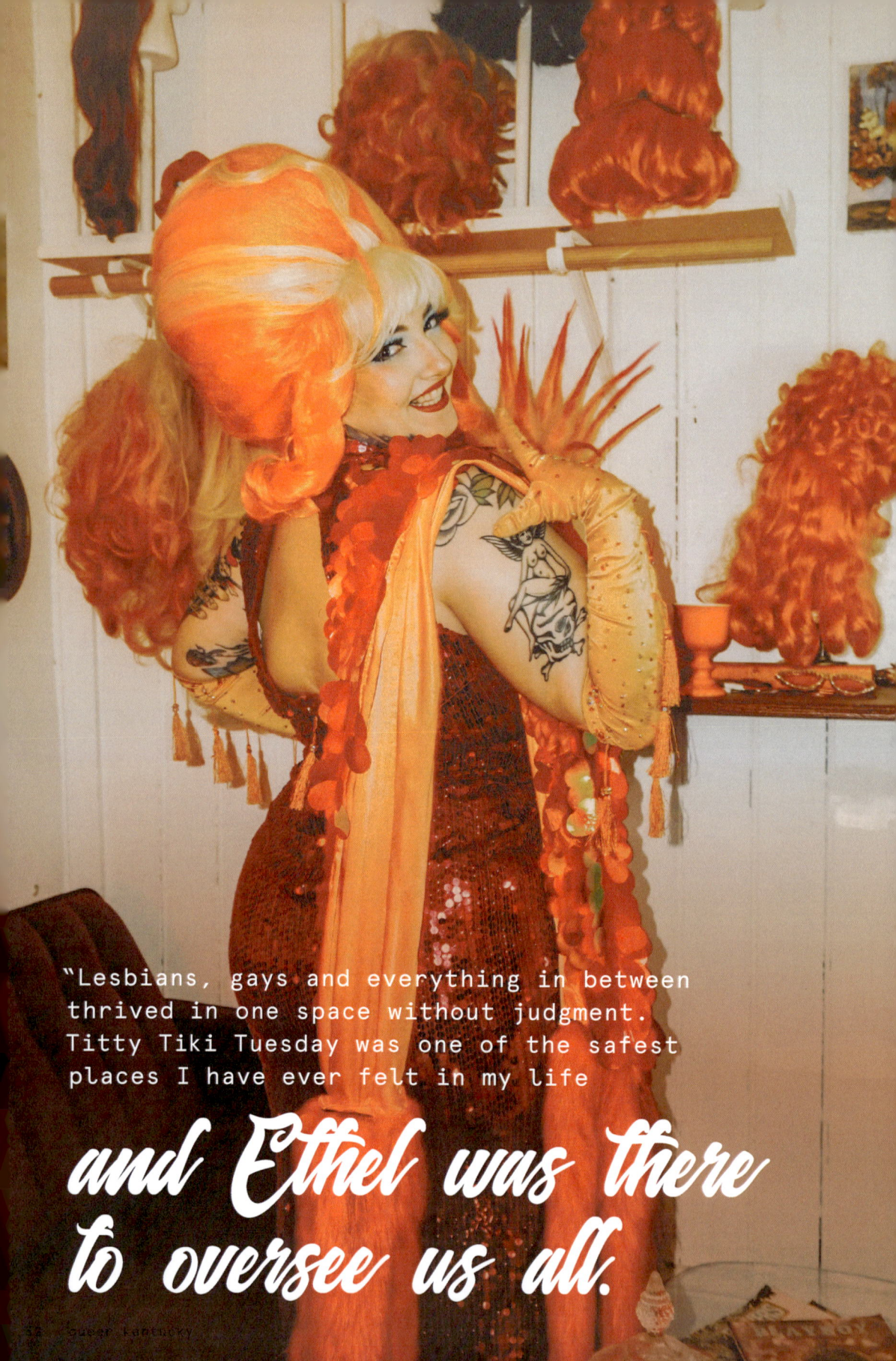

"Lesbians, gays and everything in between thrived in one space without judgment. Titty Tiki Tuesday was one of the safest places I have ever felt in my life and Ethel was there to oversee us all.

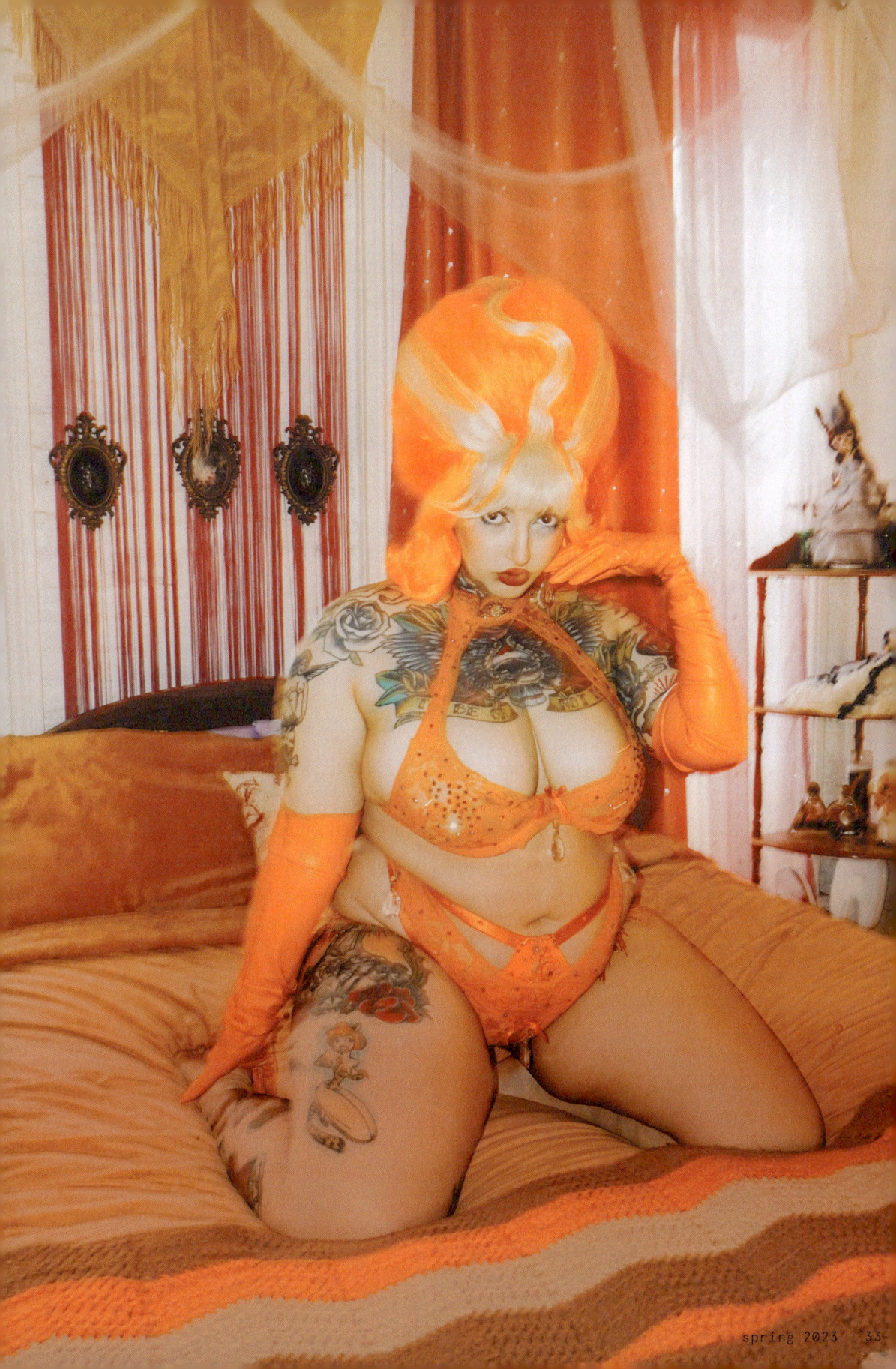

Between 2018 and 2019, I was at Titty Tiki Tuesday every week selling T-shirts to promote Queer Kentucky. The Limbo and Queer Kentucky developed a symbiotic relationship and helped market each other through our respective platforms.

I will never forget the first time I saw Ethel. She stumbled into the Limbo a bit late (diva) and a little tipsy with her bright orange wig and tasseled pasties.

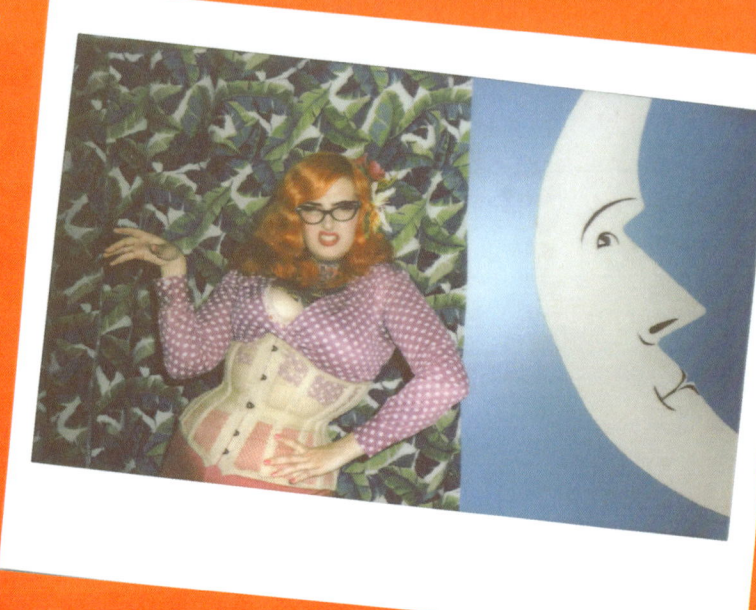

That night, while she continued painting on her face, no mirror needed, I walked up to her in my shy and eye-wandering way and asked if she could give Queer Kentucky a little shout out and tell people to come buy our shirts and learn about us.

And this doe-eyed figure took one look at me, and said, "Hey, sexy, fuck yeah, I will!"

My night was made.

Even though we had never met and she had zero idea what Queer Kentucky was, she was down to uplift my project and me just because I had asked her to. Her eagerness to help a stranger affirmed me. That is how you create community.

As the show opened and I got my shout out, I could also tell Ethel had no idea who she would be introducing and how she would be emceeing that evening, but luckily DJ Spring Break had a cheat sheet ready to go for her. This would be the first night of many I would watch the collaborative spark between the two light up an entire room.

Once Ethel took a shot and cleared her throat, the show was on! The sensual, shrilly, and mildly nasal voice welcomed everyone to a night they would never forget.

I hadn't had many queer nightlife experiences in my life until I began my journey with Queer Kentucky. I had no idea there was a community so vulgar yet so pure waiting to wrap me up in its arms. Ethel mothered me into a community every Tuesday night that year, and I'm not even sure if she knows that. I know that I am one of many that Ethel showed love and acceptance to, and I'm forever grateful.

Ethel is community.

Not only did this short moment in history set the foundation for my queerness and love for myself, but I also believe it was the foundation of a new generation of queers in Kentucky.

The Limbo and Titty Tiki Tuesday embraced the genderqueer and the curious. Trans identities weren't questioned, but celebrated. We ignored bathroom signage and existed authentically without care. Lesbians, gays and everything in between and beyond thrived in one space without judgment. Titty Tiki Tuesday was one of the safest places I have ever felt in my life, and Ethel was there looking after us.

Tuesdays were magical and I'm lucky to have lived through this little blip of queer Kentucky history.

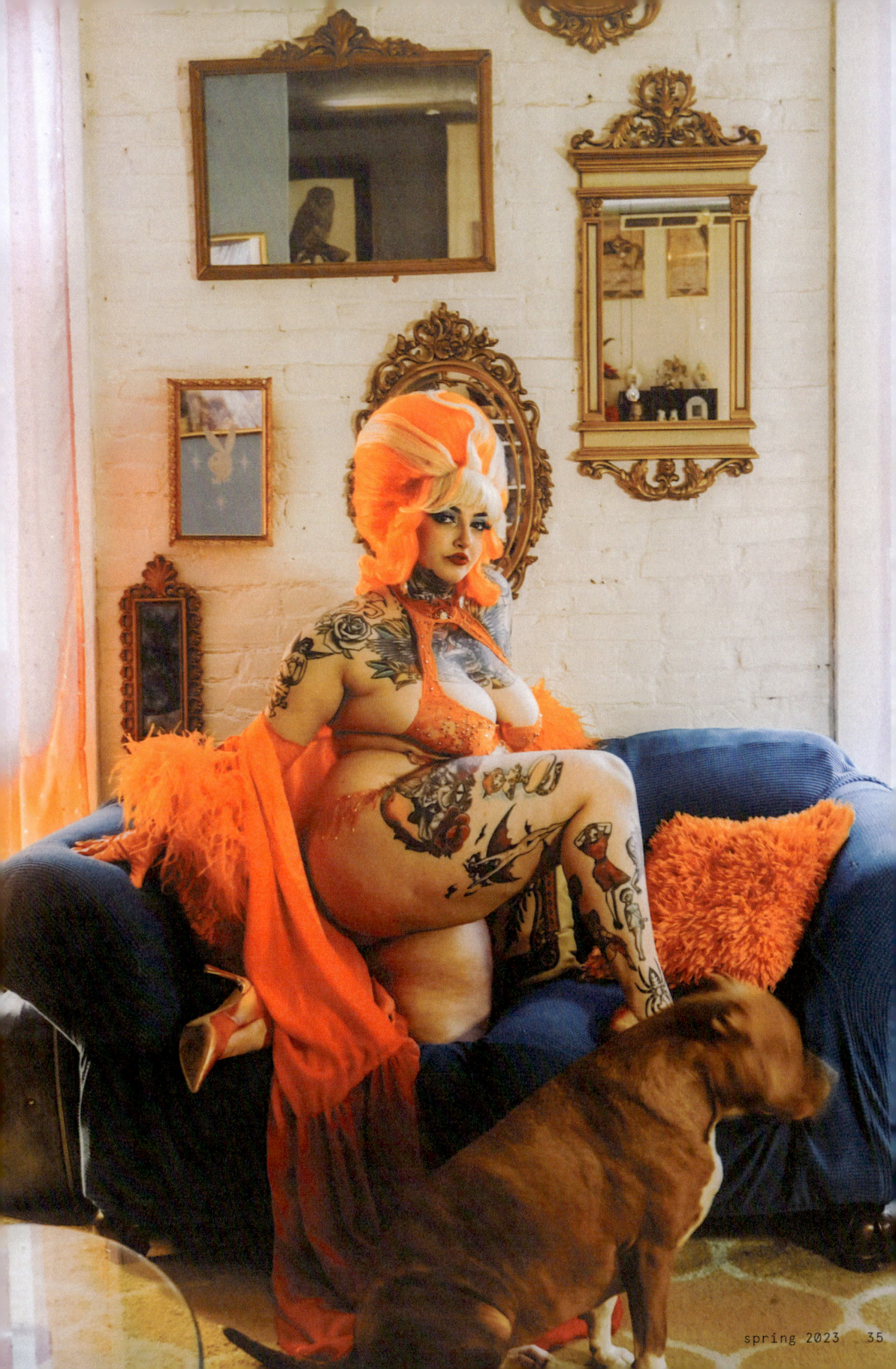

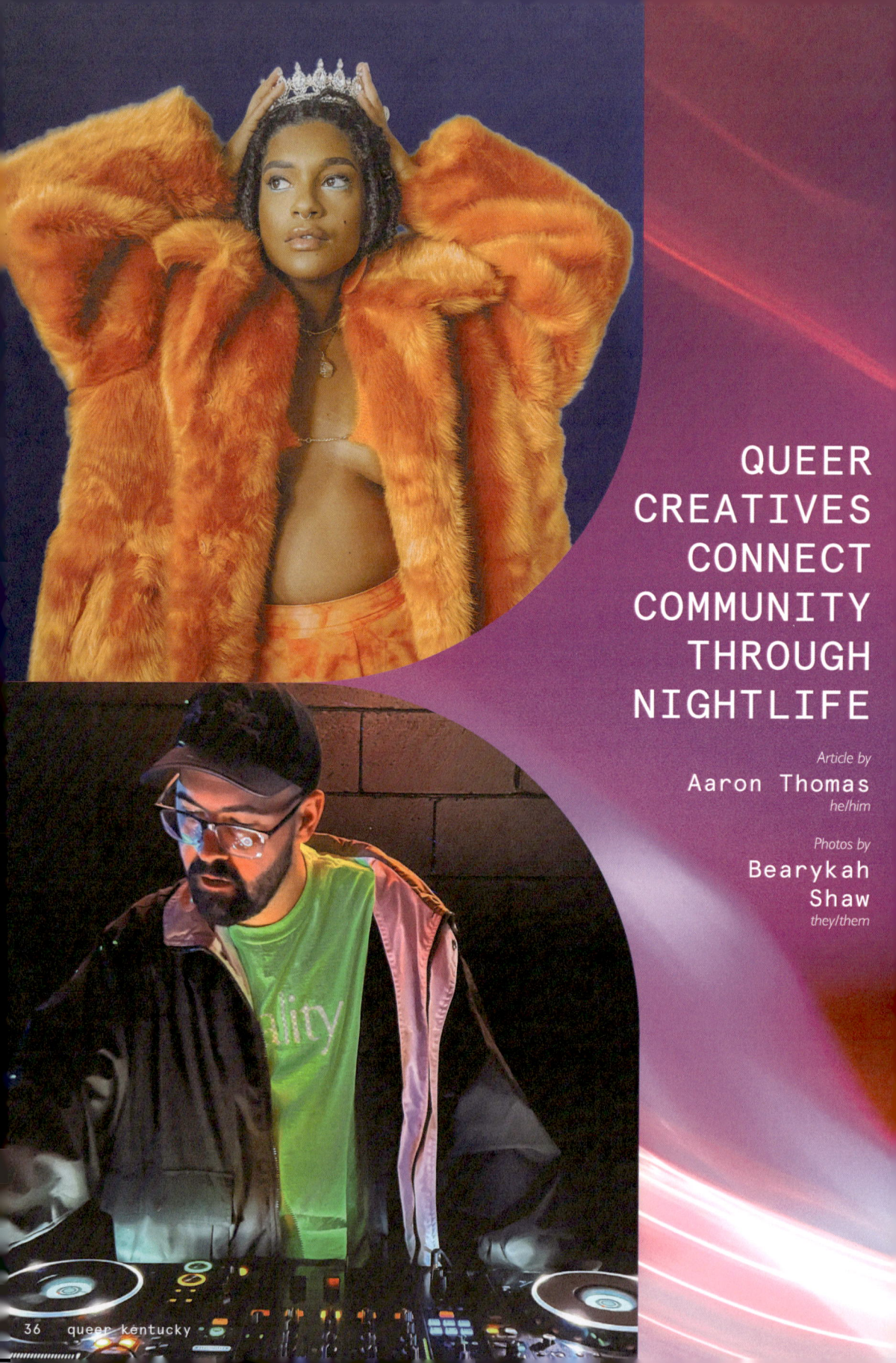

QUEER CREATIVES CONNECT COMMUNITY THROUGH NIGHTLIFE

Article by
Aaron Thomas
he/him

Photos by
Bearykah Shaw
they/them

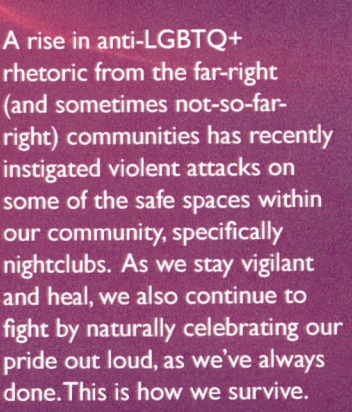

A rise in anti-LGBTQ+ rhetoric from the far-right (and sometimes not-so-far-right) communities has recently instigated violent attacks on some of the safe spaces within our community, specifically nightclubs. As we stay vigilant and heal, we also continue to fight by naturally celebrating our pride out loud, as we've always done. This is how we survive.

We've shined a spotlight on five performance artists in the Kentucky nightlife scene that have created a sense of security in these spaces for us through their craft.

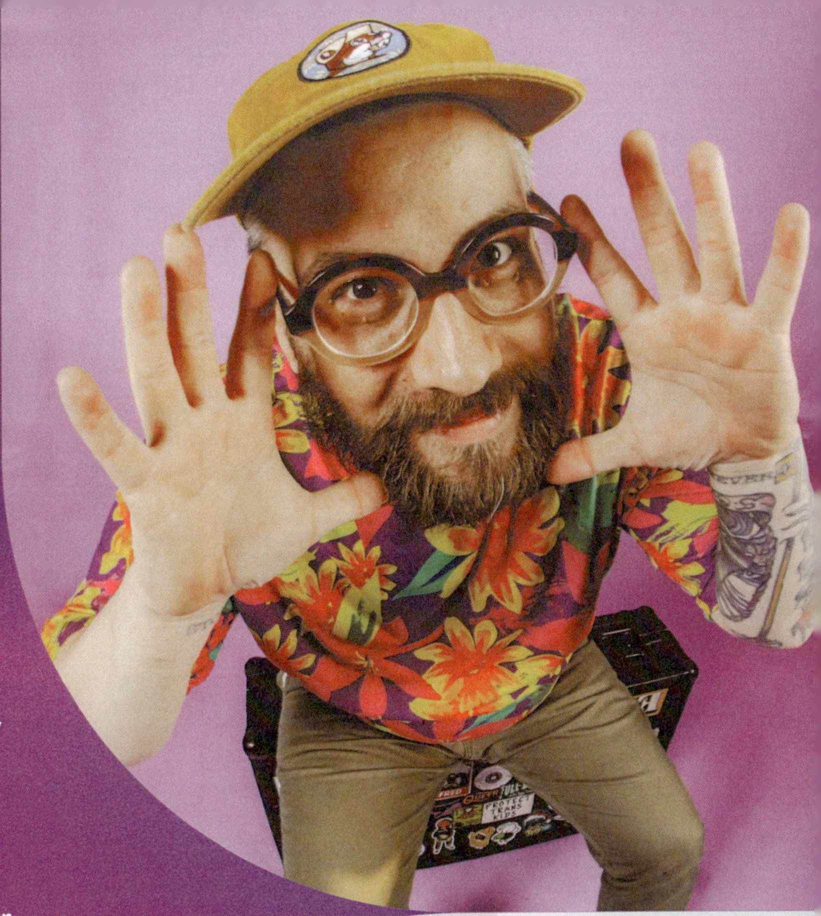

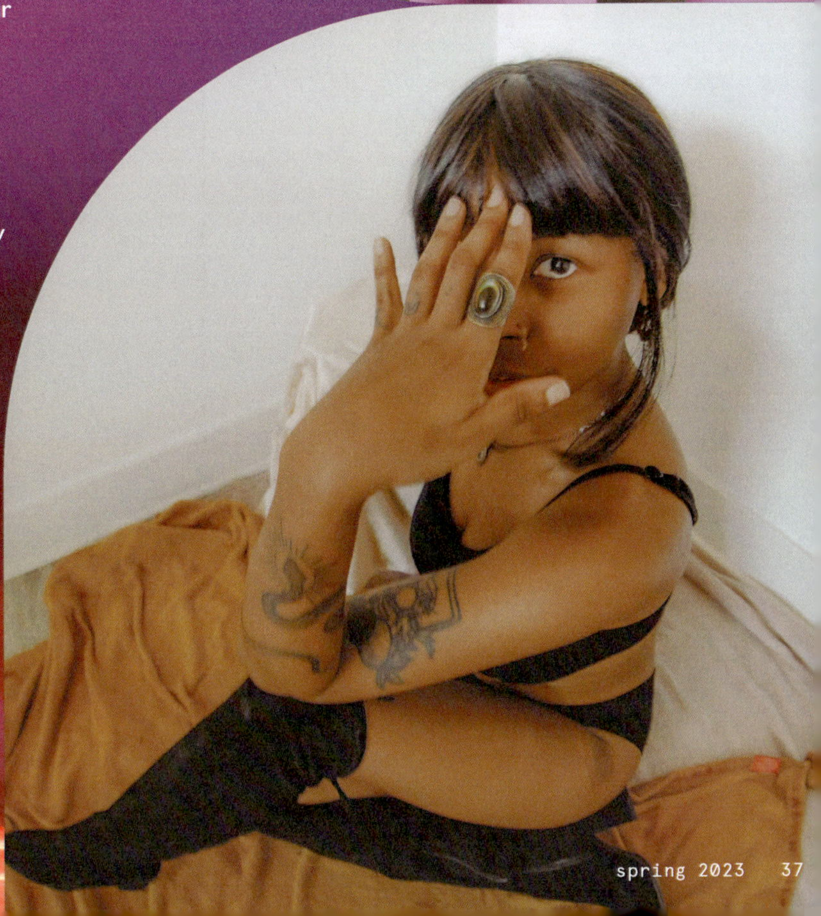

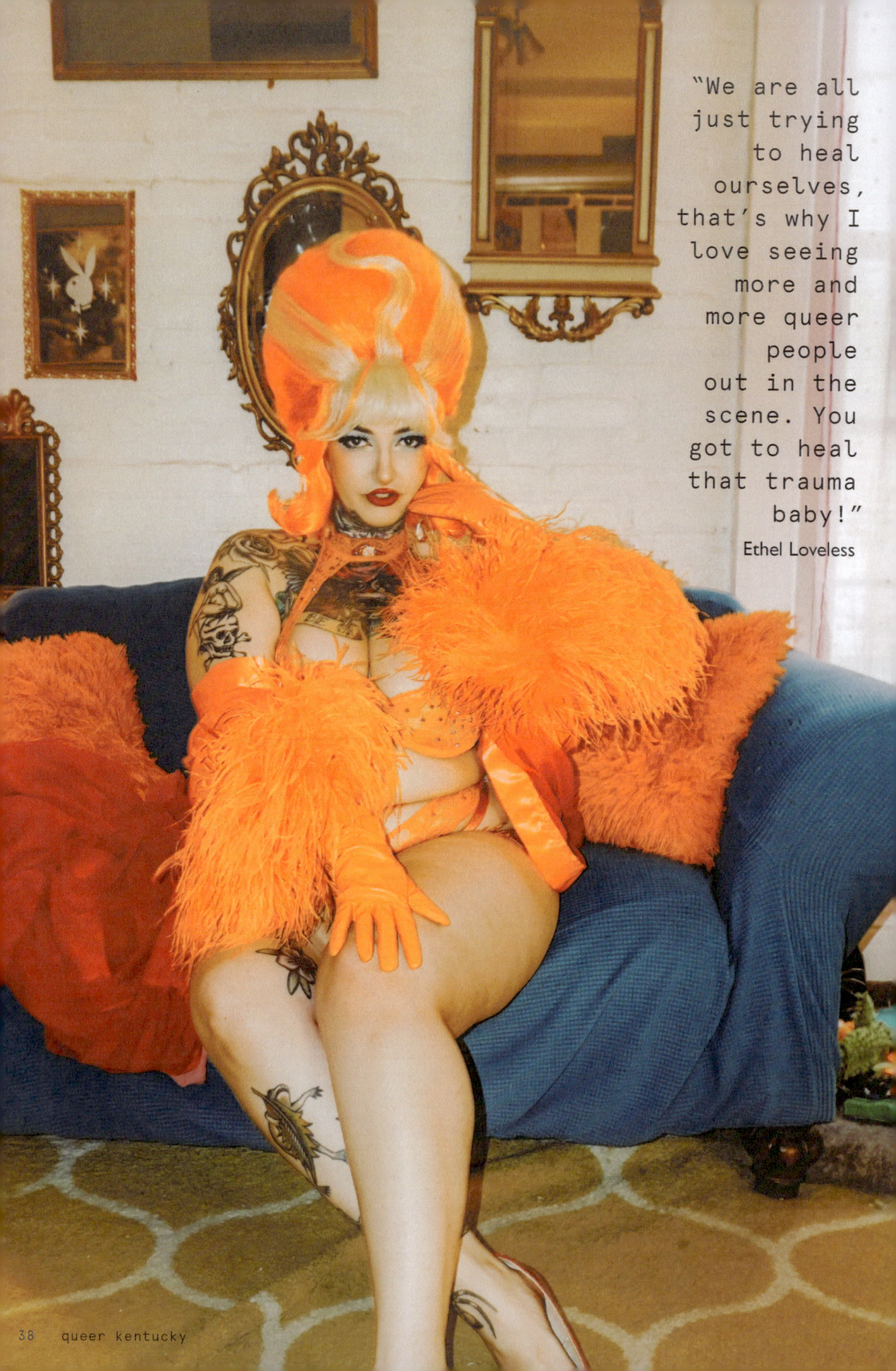

"We are all just trying to heal ourselves, that's why I love seeing more and more queer people out in the scene. You got to heal that trauma baby!"

Ethel Loveless

ETHEL LOVELESS

Self-proclaimed "Traveling Tangerine Showgirl"

(she/they)

I left my hometown of Bardstown when I was 17 or 18 years old because I've always felt this fire inside of me that I wanted to add oil to. I saw my first burlesque show shortly after and was like "Holy shit, this is my awakening." I then began the process of making my Moulin Rouge fantasy from when I was six years old a reality.

The world I know now is a collective community of clown/punk/sleazy/cute/messy/beautiful people. It's become my life and my family and I love it all.

I've learned to express myself as me and just see people for who they are without having those restrictions that normal small-town life can have on you.

The empowerment of burlesque dancing comes from how normal and natural it feels, yet it's so taboo in society. I know it's not normal for everyone but my community is so open and kind. We want you to feel empowered, but you're gonna have to work for it. Confidence comes from within. We can't teach you that part.

It's very important for all people, but especially queer people, to feel safe. Even if they are getting "ead" across the bar, I want them to feel safe. These spaces shouldn't be limited to queer-produced events or establishments only. I want to see more mainstream commercial spaces accept and therefore begin to normalize queer culture.

There are so many nasty people that want to hurt the people I love. And I hate that. It makes me frazzled.

TIGRESSE BLEU

Dancer, poet, mystic, and artist

(she/they)

What I'm really doing is reading energy. Tarot and crystals are just tools. I find energy in anything: tea leaves, coffee grounds, dirt, literally anything. It's all purely intuitive and satisfying for me as someone who likes to work with their hands.

It wasn't necessarily about doing burlesque. I had heard of it but never knew what it all entailed. I just wanted to dance. I always feel better and grounded when I can move my body.

I've experienced a lot by just getting out there and doing it. Just diving in and saying, "fuck it", then learning as I go.

Through dancing and other forms of arts, I get to share with my community, I only feel closer to myself.

Anytime I've ever stepped into a performance, I've always felt at home. You don't get that everywhere. I'm so happy I've had the opportunity to be amongst other people who strive to cultivate a space where others can be free in themselves safely. That's all any of us in the queer art scene want.

There's a reason studying astrology has been around for thousands of years. I love taking a horoscope and making it better, more queer-friendly if you will. I find that a lot of the language is outdated and thinks of things in a strict binary. People feeling included and understood through my writings on astrology is also very important.

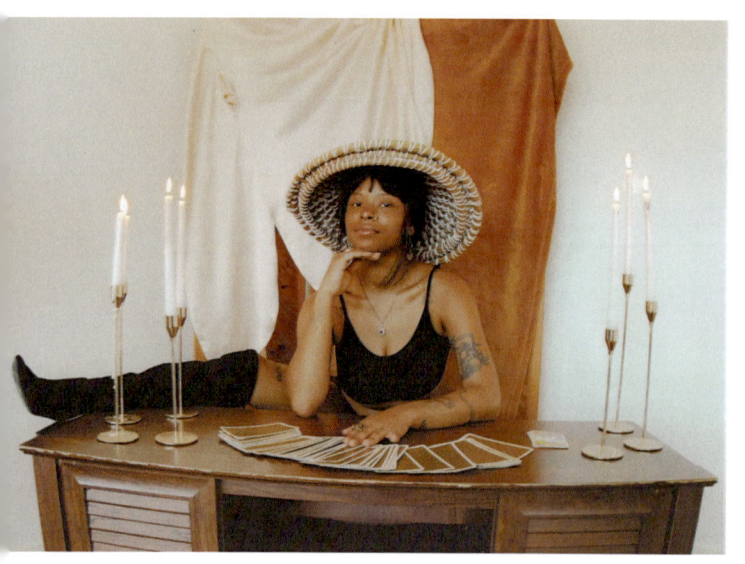

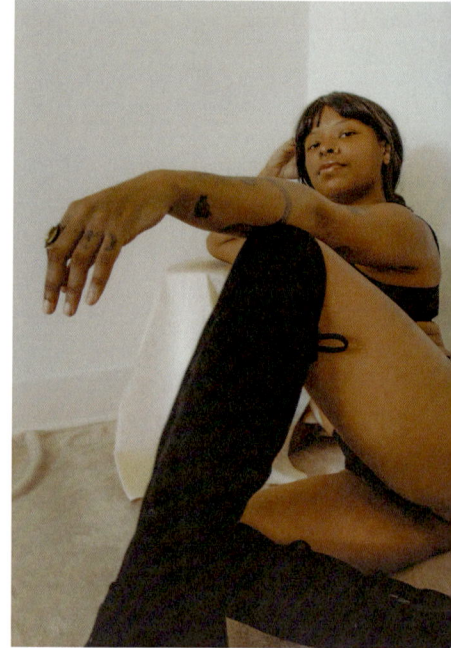

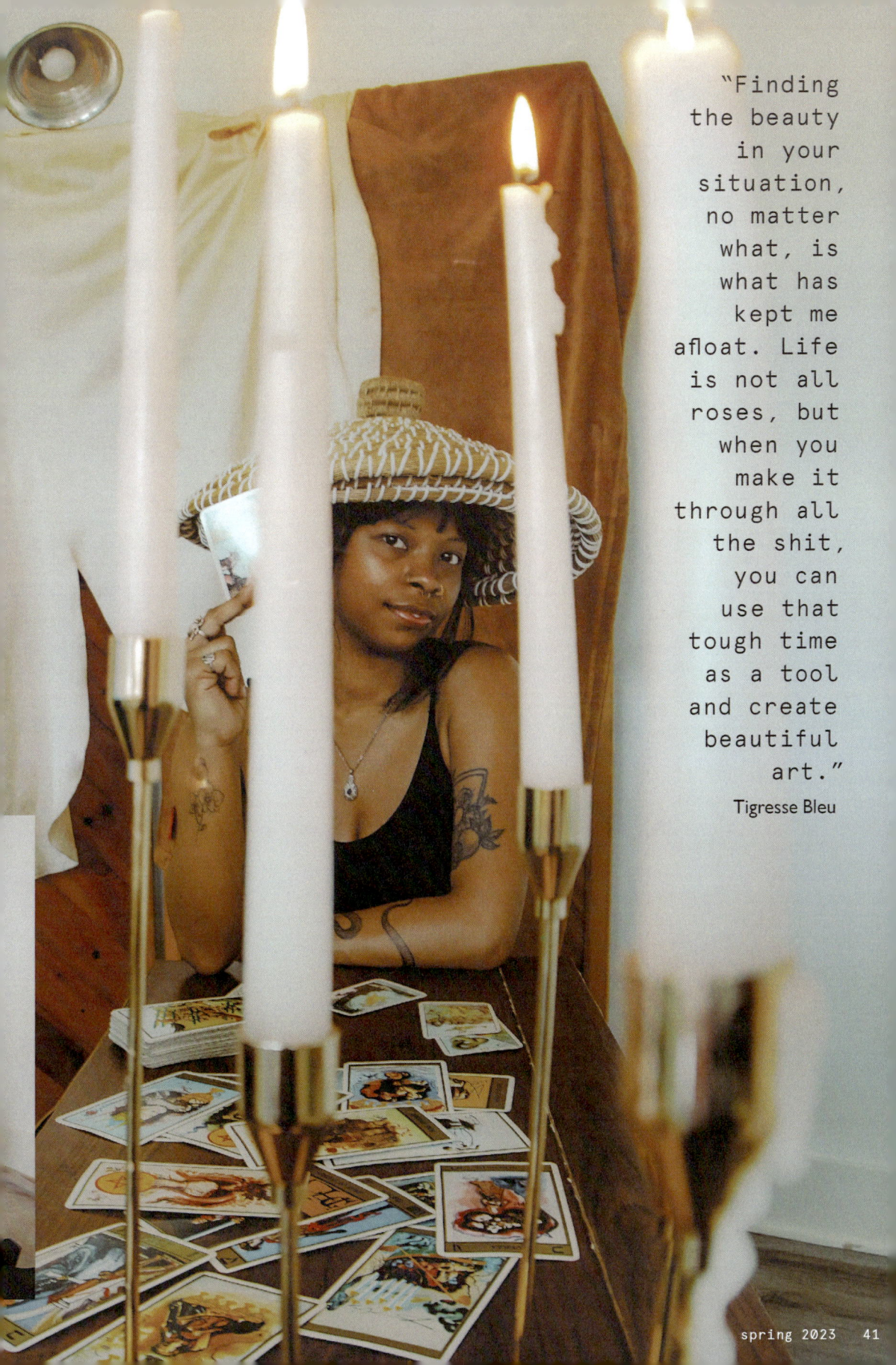

"Finding the beauty in your situation, no matter what, is what has kept me afloat. Life is not all roses, but when you make it through all the shit, you can use that tough time as a tool and create beautiful art."

Tigresse Bleu

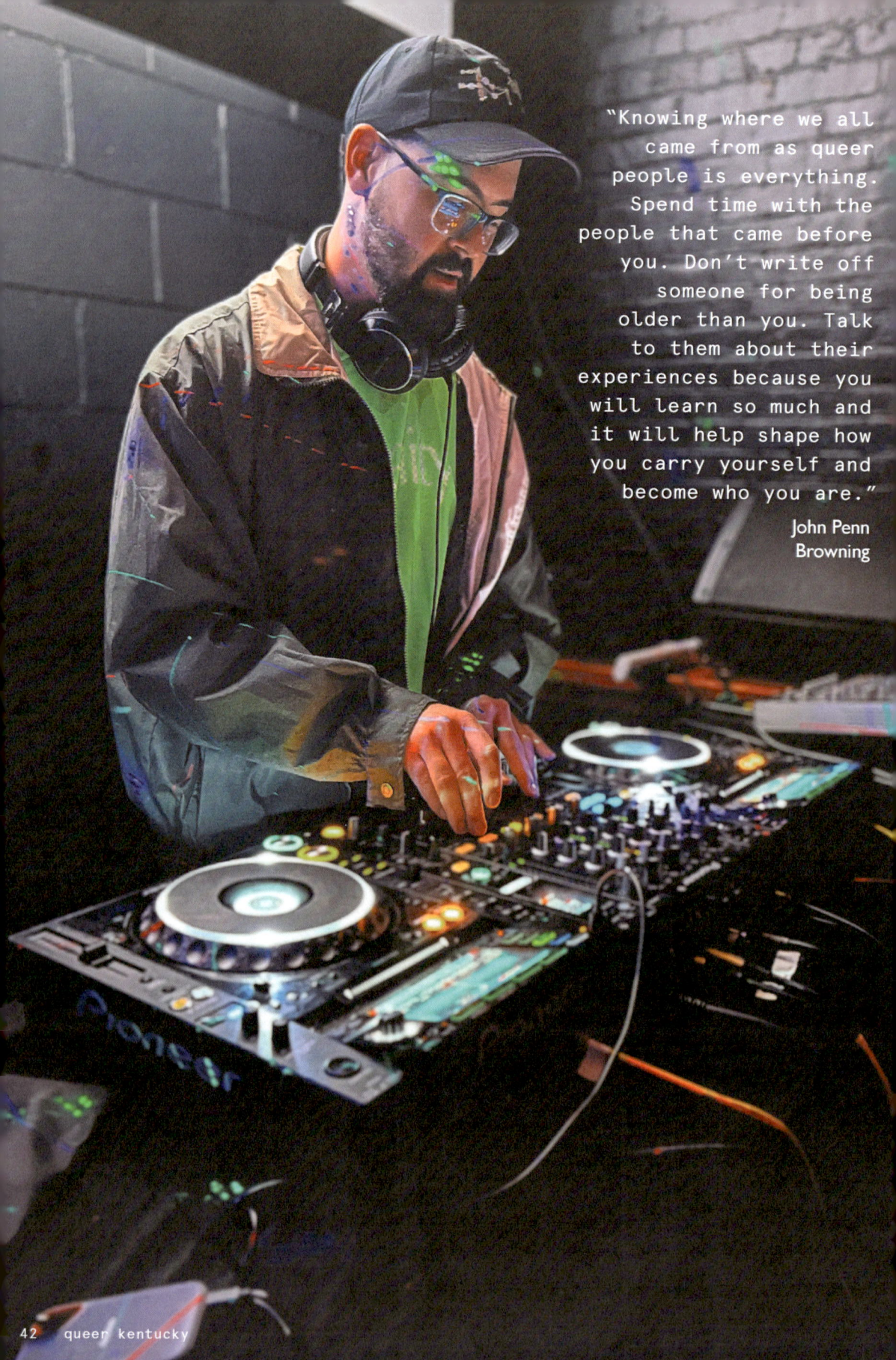

"Knowing where we all came from as queer people is everything. Spend time with the people that came before you. Don't write off someone for being older than you. Talk to them about their experiences because you will learn so much and it will help shape how you carry yourself and become who you are."

John Penn Browning

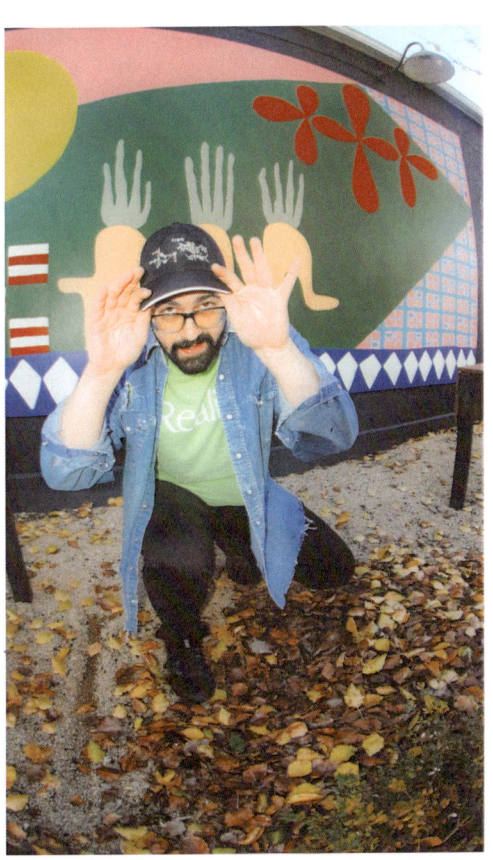

JOHN PENN BROWNING

DJ, dance music enthusiast, and self-described "amateur" bartender

(he/him)

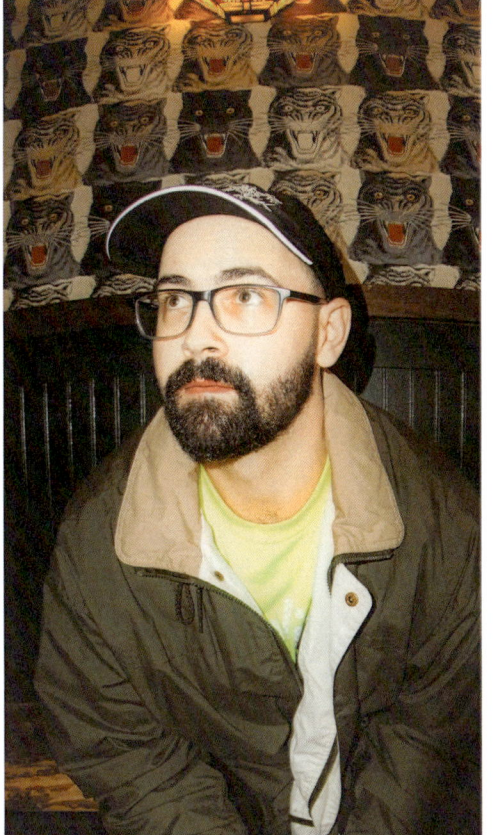

I love the rush of discovering something inspiring that I can share with people and watching them just vibe with it.

Empowering your music community is the groundwork. You have to make sure that people know you're paying attention. Remind them that you see and hear the effort they are putting into their crafts. That's super important.

As far back as I can remember, I've always been on the hunt for music. I mean I fucking loved it. I was raised around a lot of hip-hop and that influences the soul I love so much with disco.

I know my general appearance can kind of fall under the radar sometimes in many spaces. Especially with the artistry of DJing and the knowledge that goes behind that, you have the power to exude the safeness in the space with the music you are playing.

DESTINY CARTER

Musician, DJ DNasti, multi-media artist, radio host, community activist, flow artist, curator

(she/her)

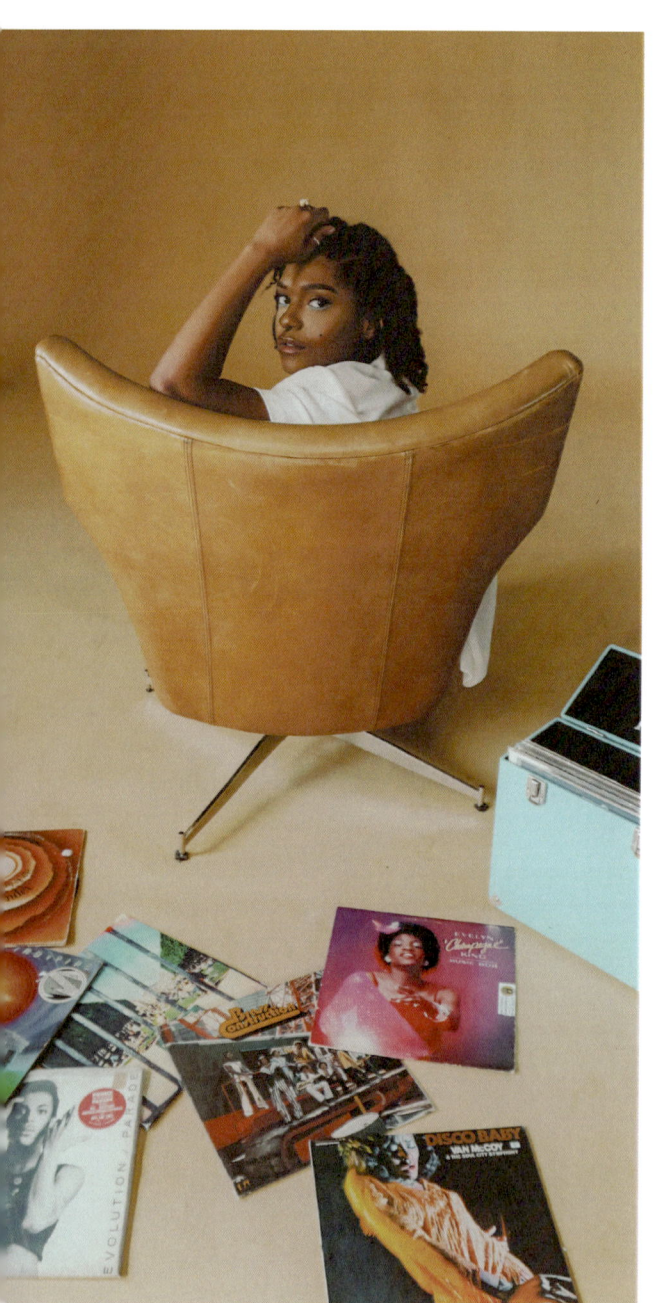

Individualism is pushed a lot and there's no point in me getting to a place where everyone around me is still somewhere else. Success for me is all of us getting to a place we can freely create and freely be ourselves together in one space unapologetically.

I am a teacher and a motivator in my community. I get it: these bigger cities have more opportunities, but if all of my fellow queer creatives leave Kentucky, who is going to keep that creative impact going while they are gone? There will be nothing to come back to.

Just existing in the world as a black queer woman has always had some type of hesitation in many spaces, but we're also pioneers and leaders. Arriving as myself, not as a "token", is a representation in itself. But, I also want to make sure my identity as a black queer woman is always heard, and therefore make sure everyone who feels underrepresented is heard as well.

I was introduced to the queer community growing up through a white male lens, so knowing who you are in your own skin is queerness in itself because it's coming from you.

Who is showing up in the world is for us and at the end of the day, that is our personal expression, so we can't let anyone take that from us.

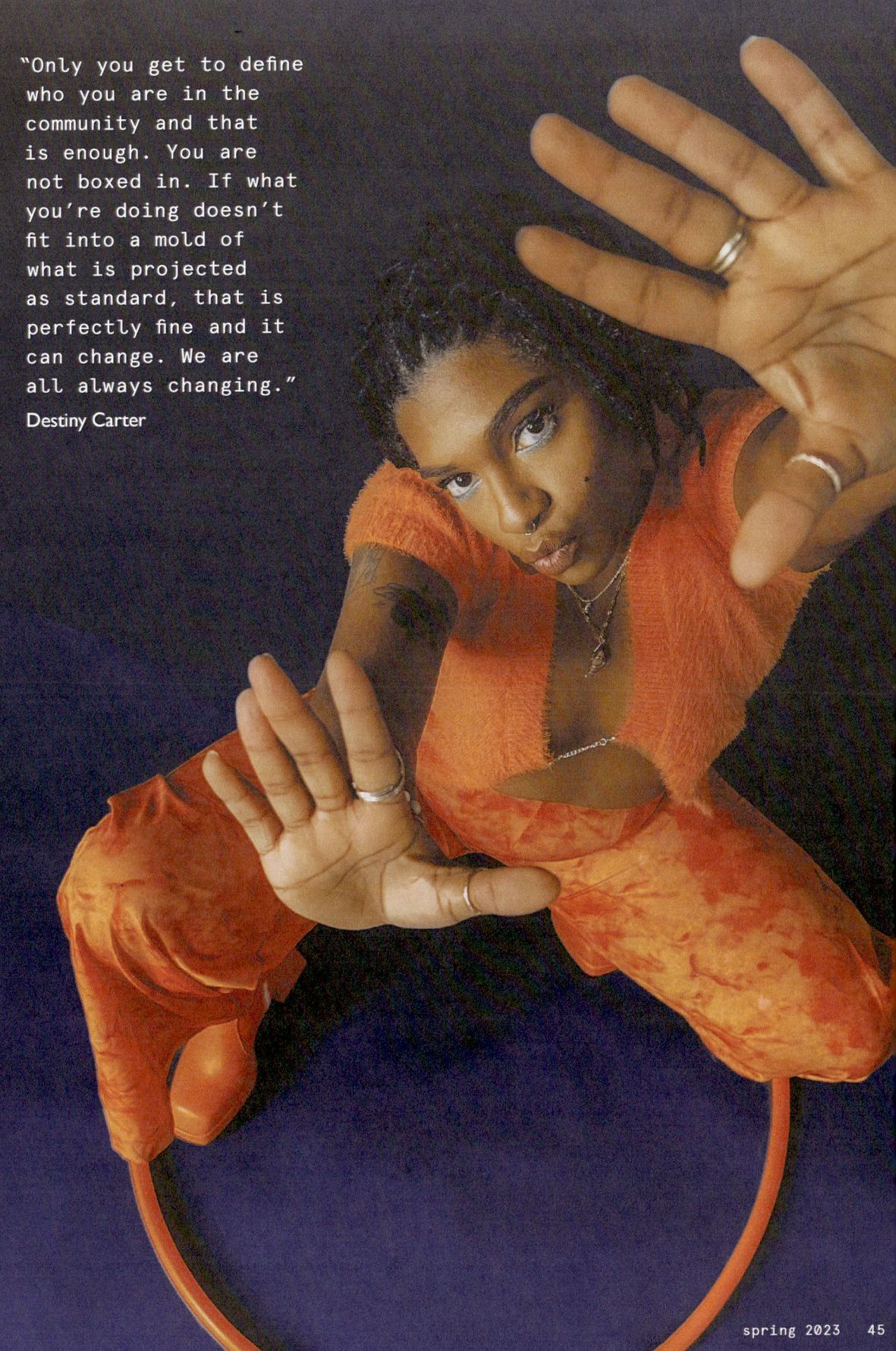

"Only you get to define who you are in the community and that is enough. You are not boxed in. If what you're doing doesn't fit into a mold of what is projected as standard, that is perfectly fine and it can change. We are all always changing."
Destiny Carter

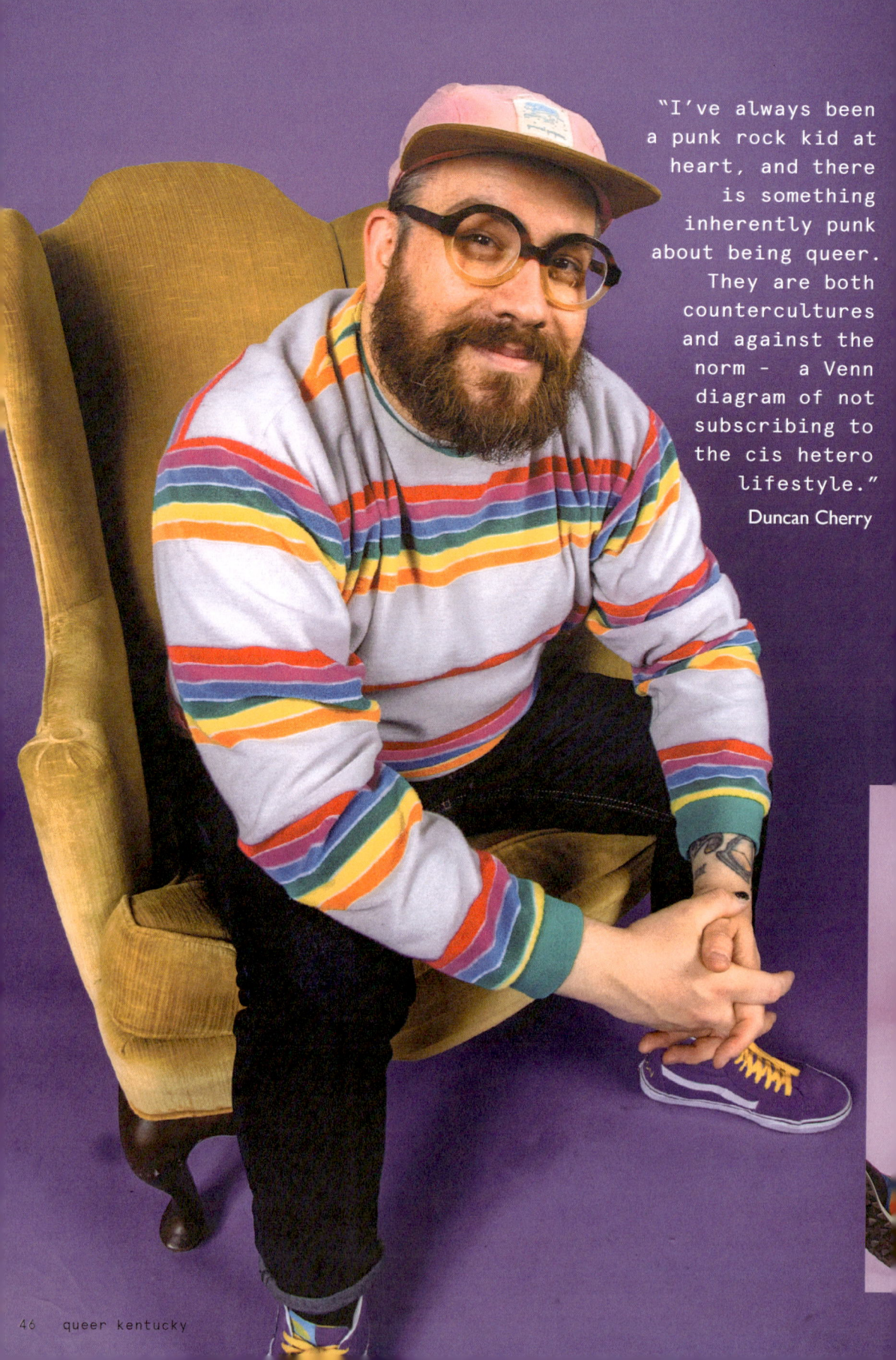

"I've always been a punk rock kid at heart, and there is something inherently punk about being queer. They are both countercultures and against the norm - a Venn diagram of not subscribing to the cis hetero lifestyle."
Duncan Cherry

DUNCAN CHERRY

DJ Spring Break,
curator, co-producer

(he/him)

DJing came from the hustle a.k.a. the do-it-yourself culture. It's my thing, my world, and what I can do to create an environment, atmosphere, and aesthetic that is purely me.

As a community, are we keeping ourselves safe as a unit? There is a level of care and awareness that comes with being queer. Like, we have to look out for one another because no one else is going to do those things for us.

We are not on a baseball team, you know? Sports figures get praised constantly, but queer artists doing incredible things with the highest of heels and the highest of hair get ignored, or even worse, shamed because they are deemed "weird."

Being queer has always been perceived as different. It's where we fall in, but it's where we fall together.

The most important thing you can do is to find your people. Finding others who are like you is a reminder that you are not alone.

Our accents of uniqueness are what make us special. People will tell you you're weird, you're different, and that you'll never fit in. But, it is all of those things that make you stand out in a crowd.

My meaning of life is to be a magnet and to connect through things I am magnetized to. That's how our community is built.

We are a never-ending pyramid. Our elders at the base have laid the groundwork and the top is ours to build up towards and the sky is the absolute limit.

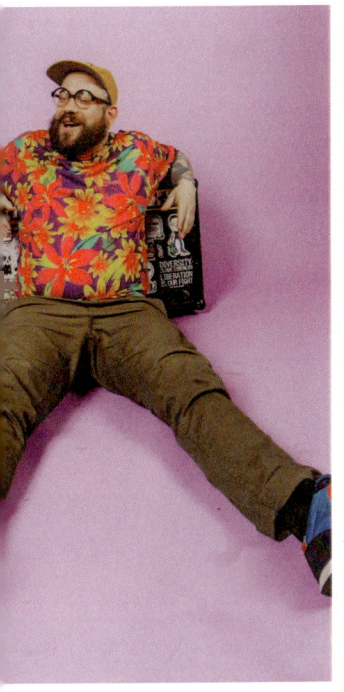
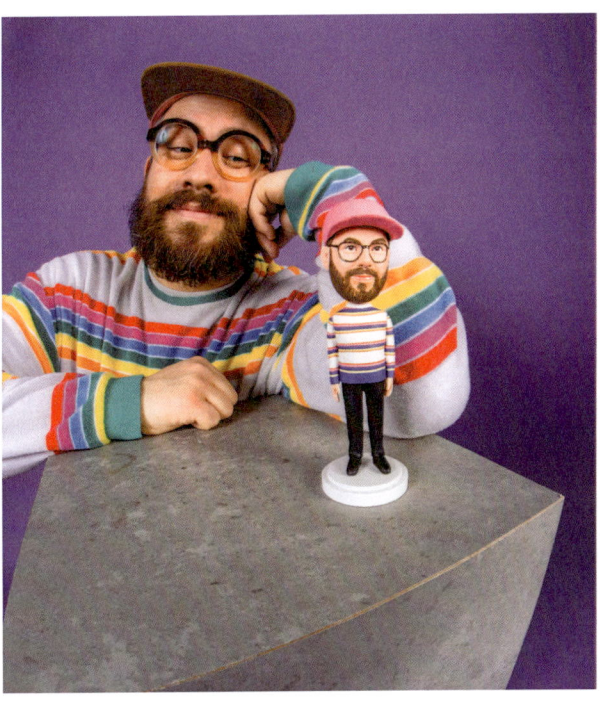

The Trevor Project
estimates that more than

1.8 MILLION

LGBTQ youth (13-24)
seriously consider suicide
each year in the U.S.

At least one
attempts suicide

EVERY 45 SECONDS

Get help or learn more
www.thetrevorproject.org

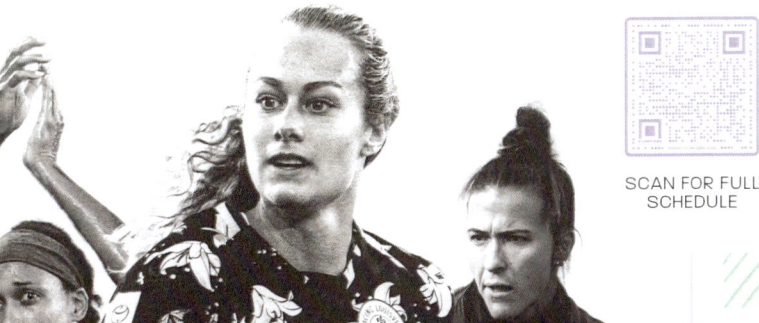
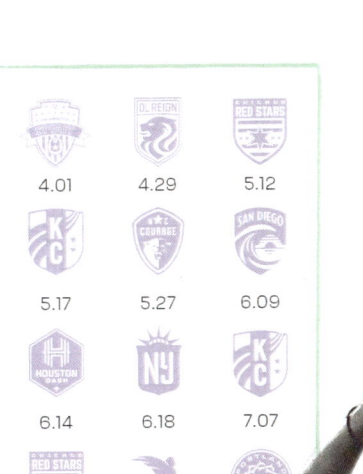
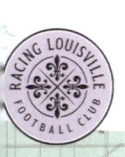
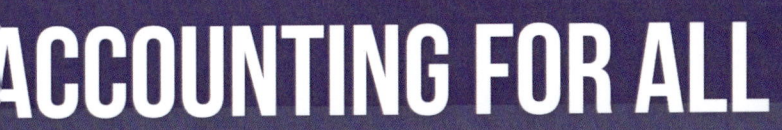

Are Therapists Sufficiently Trained to Help LGBTQ+ Clients?

Emma Koenig *she/her*

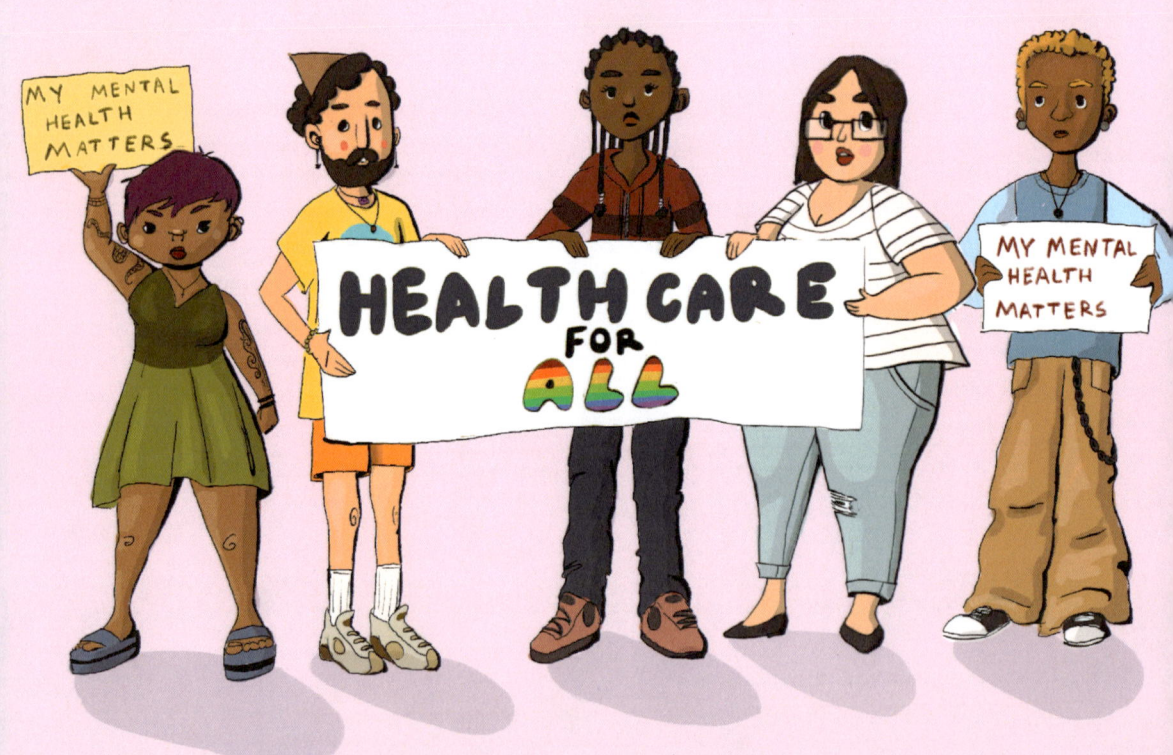

Artwork by Betty Agajyelleh *she/her*

Mental healthcare continues to be inequitable for LGBTQ+ identifying individuals, despite the community's disproportionate need. Members of minority groups are unlikely to seek therapy, largely as a result of inadequate education on these communities' unique mental health needs, as well as a lack of diversity (Burgess, 2008; Clark, 2004). Such issues have led to ineffective, and therefore undesirable, therapy for LGBTQ+ community members.

"Mental health and healthcare in general has overlooked LGBTQ+ people for generations. Many of the professionals I was working alongside didn't quite know how to help LGBTQ people and therefore had to be okay with the bare minimum," says Robert Kyle May, owner of Open Doors Counseling Center in Kentucky.

In addition to the financial, societal, and professional inequality which affects LGBTQ+ people's access to mental healthcare, "many members of minority groups feel that therapists (many of whom identify with the majority, even today) would be unable to understand their lived experiences and fully address their needs."

Intersectionalities in these communities combine and compound, making mental healthcare even less accessible. While 42% of the American LGBTQ+ community is non-white, only 17% of the U.S. psychology workforce are. This leaves many minority groups working with therapists they do not relate to.

Dr. Joanna Morse, a Kentucky Psychologist, says she sees graduate programs becoming more knowledgeable and teaching more on client diversity, but asks, "For people who graduated years ago, how are they supposed to get up to speed?". When Dr. Morse first started working with transgender clients without specific training, she felt unprepared, learned as she went along, relied on help from her clients, and remembered it as "not feeling great for either party."

All ten Kentucky mental health professionals interviewed agreed unanimously on the lack of diversity they were exposed to in schooling and how it affected their ability to treat diverse clientele. Although there have been improvements in recent years, with sensitivity workshops and LGBTQ+ care conferences, clients still often teach the unfamiliar therapist how to give affirming care.

Robin Herrington, a Kentucky licensed counselor, shared that they were often the only openly nonbinary student in their master's classes, and when they asked specific questions about treating LGBTQ+ clients, neither the professors nor the professors' leadership could provide answers.

"Representation matters. Seeing yourself matters. Having professors that are therapists, who work with queer people matters," Harrington said.

Each Kentucky therapist interviewed stated that they received very little, if any, training or education on LGBTQ+ clients in their master's program. Not one of the professionals reported feeling sufficiently prepared to assist LGBTQ+ clients with their mental health needs after graduation. They had to independently seek out and self-teach about LGBTQ+ communities' varying mental health needs. This top-down lack of experience results in microaggressions, insensitivities, and other discourtesies which hinder the client-therapist rapport.

Jasmine Skye, a client who is biracial, pansexual, nonbinary, and autistic, states their experience of getting any type of healthcare "is a constant hell of navigating the system, even with somewhat adequate health insurance."

Many therapists I reached out to denied being interviewed as they did not feel adequately knowledgeable about equity for LGBTQ+ clients… yet they are advertising their practices as LGBTQ+ friendly and are currently working with queer folks.

An increase in healthcare access would help undo the longstanding healthcare deterrence, disparities, and discriminations that LGBTQ+ communities experience. Equal mental healthcare would go beyond improving the lives of LGBTQ+ groups. Improved access to mental healthcare would make communities safer, happier, more productive, and more united. But until that point, please use the following information to learn more about what you can do.

As an LGBTQ+ member in need of mental healthcare:

| Lean on organizations like Queer Kentucky and Open Door Counseling Center to assist with navigating mental healthcare and provide educational resources. | Reach out to healthcare providers that are willing to discuss their experience working with LGBTQ+ clients, training they've had, and use sliding scale pricing to find care within your budget. | When choosing a therapist, remember that they work for you. Feel empowered to schedule a consultation call, and ask specific questions about what affirming care means to them, or about their particular journey to becoming an affirming therapist to ensure that you feel comfortable and safe speaking with them. | Remember you can stop working with a therapist if you ever feel uncomfortable or unaffirmed. |

As a mental health professional:

| Seek outside training, conferences, and workshops to independently learn to better treat people from minority groups. | Push back and ask questions to educators and speakers in school, work, and training sessions about minority groups to bring awareness to areas of weakness the institutions may still have. | Allow clients to ask questions, schedule consultation calls, and approach the relationship slowly to gain trust and comfort. |

| Be loud and proud about who you treat and who you are accepting of. Seeing and hearing that you're proud of treating LGBTQ+ clients allows them to trust that you walk the walk. | If you feel underqualified to treat someone based on their identity, be upfront about this until you've gained better insight/education. Until then, do your best to build out a referral network of other providers they might be able to see instead. |

As an ally:

| If you're able to, donate money, time, or resources to organizations in your area that help LGBTQ+ individuals to access better mental healthcare services. | Be there to support your friends and family in navigating the mental healthcare system, as it can be frustrating and discouraging. Offer to help in whatever ways they may need, and be patient. | Attend and show support for local LGBTQ+ events held in your community. |

Biblo

Burgess, D.J., Ding, Y., Hargreaves, M., Van Ryn, M., & Phelan, S. (2008). The association between perceived discrimination and underutilization of needed medical health care in a multi-ethnic community sample. *Journal of Health Care for the Poor and Underserved, 19*(3), 894-911. doi:10.1353/hpu.0.0063

Clark, E.J. (2004). Health disparities: Social workers helping communities move from statistics to solutions. Retrieved from: http://www.socialworkers.org/pressroom/2004/040804b.asp

Herrington emphasized that everyone needs to "Do the work, too. Try harder. Be part of the community. Educate yourself. And do all the things" to make room for everyone in the mental healthcare space.

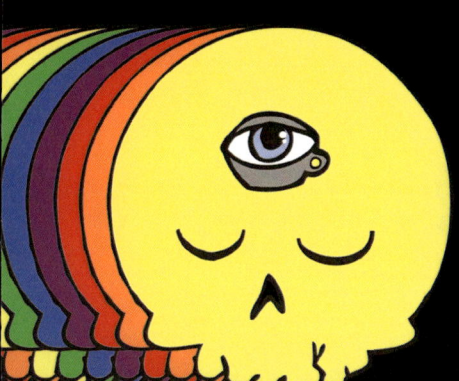

LUSSI BROWN COFFEE BAR

EST. 2017

LUSSIBROWNCOFFEE.COM

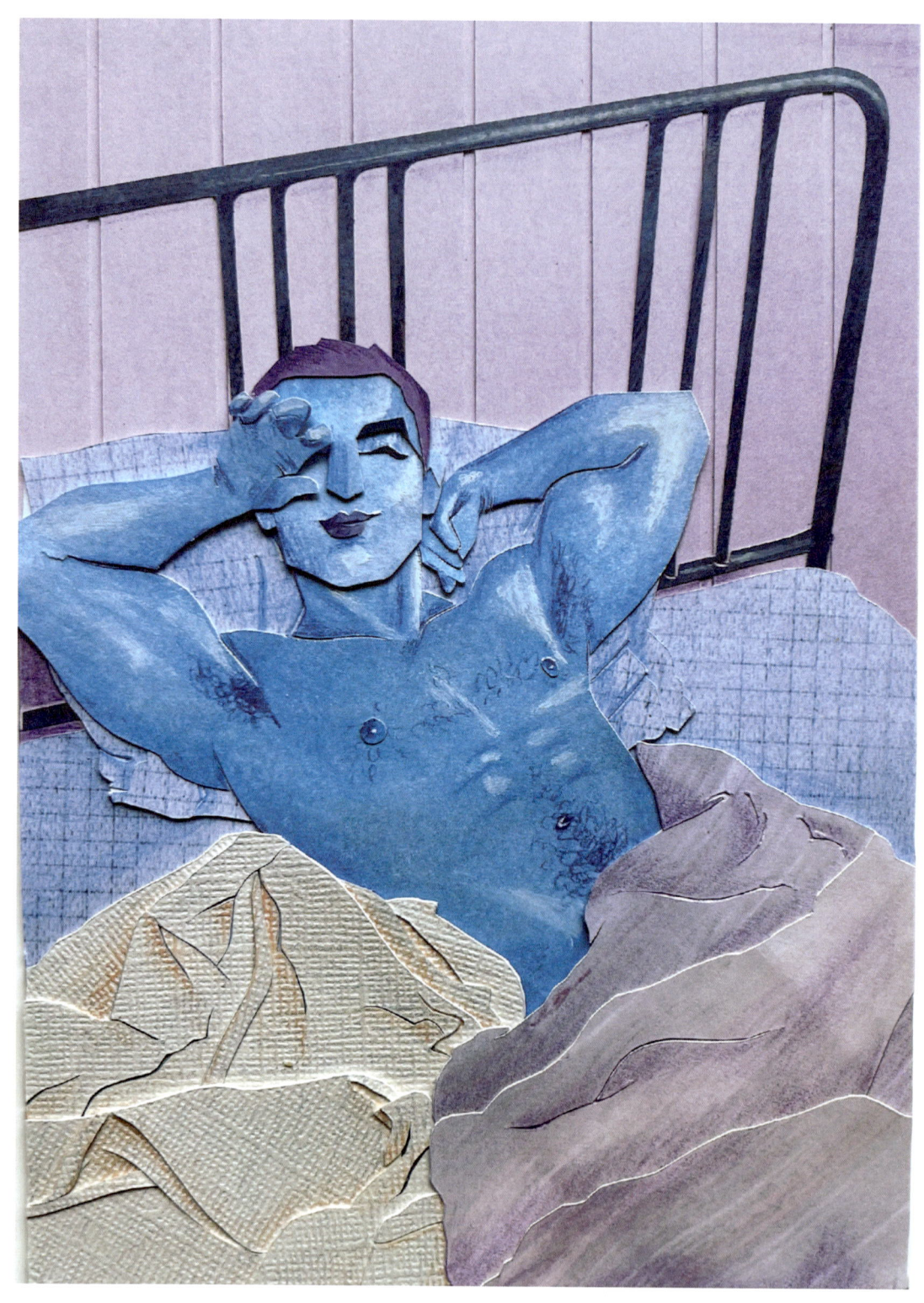

MINIATURE PORTRAITS
Jack Manion *he/him*

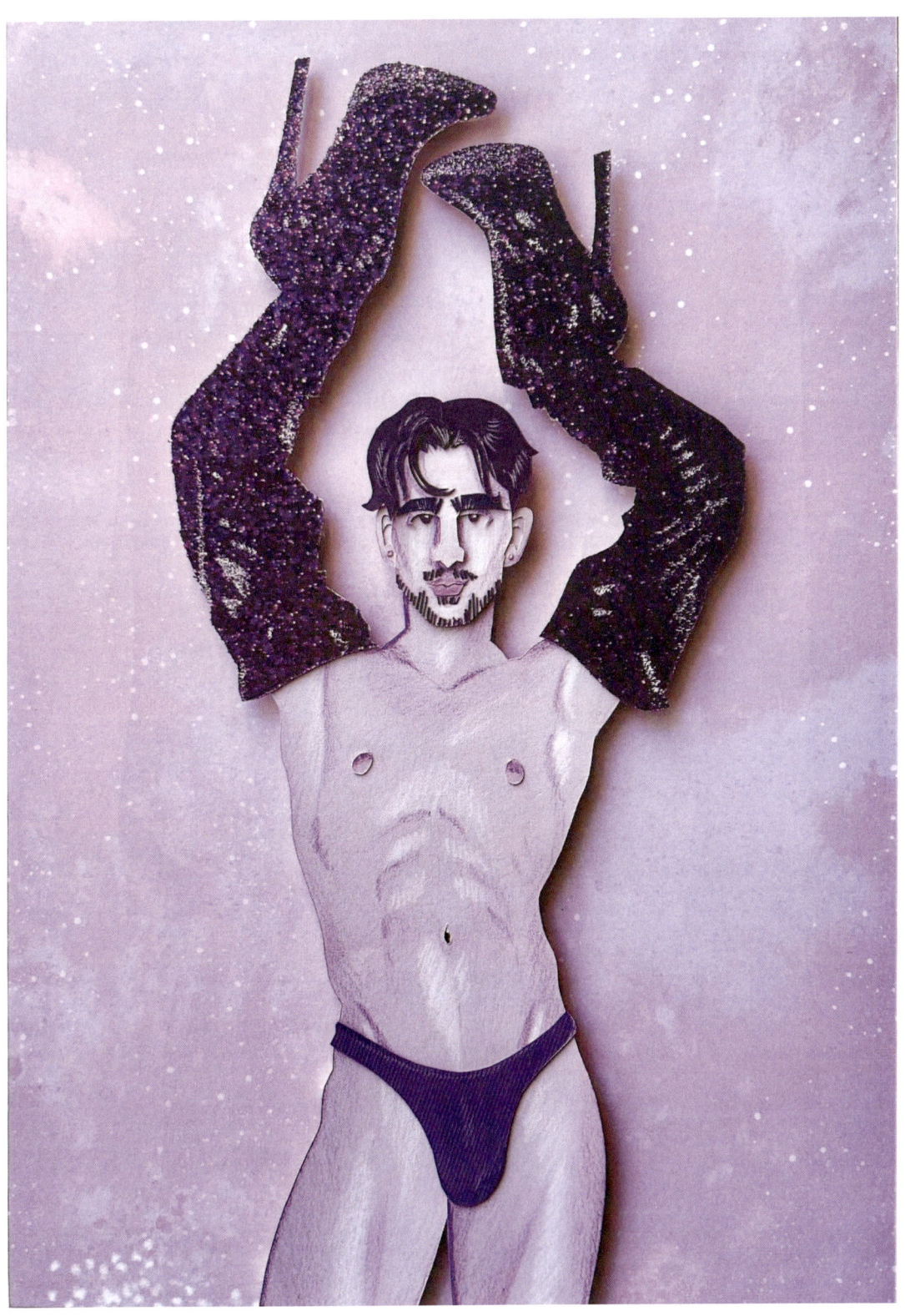

Access to Trans-Healthcare with Kellee Duke

Sydni Hampton
they/them, she/her

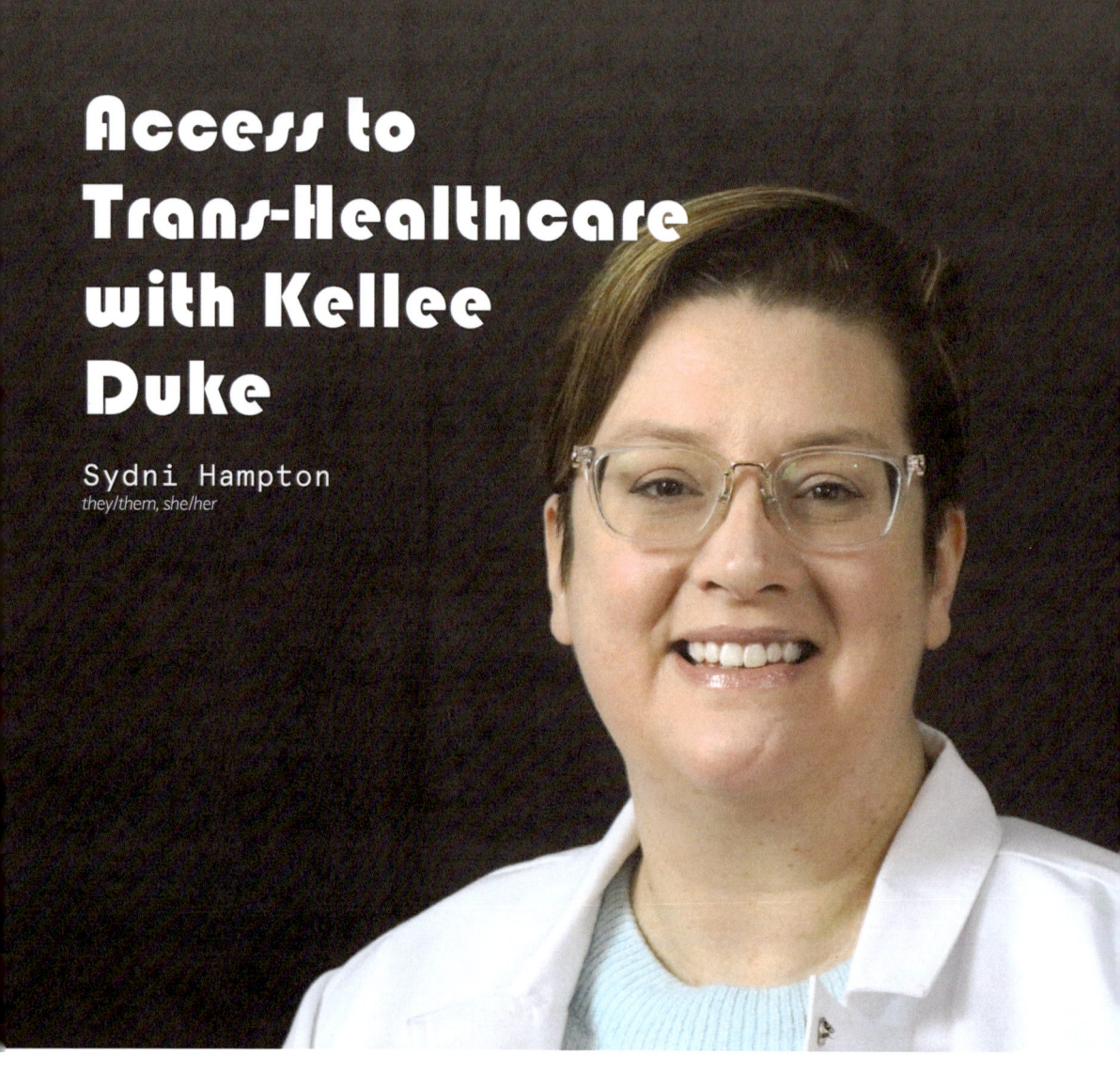

In 2023, trans affirming healthcare is available and affordable, but many wonder where to begin. I asked The Family Health Center's Kellee Duke (she/her), MSN, APRN, FNP-BC, to share information to shed some light surrounding trans-affirming healthcare. FHC is a community health center whose mission is to provide access to high quality primary and preventive healthcare services without regard to the ability to pay.

Photo from University of Louisville

Sydni: What would be the first step getting started with HRT, should someone wish to medically transition?

Kellee: I think the first step is to find a primary care provider that you trust and have a good relationship with. This can be a challenge, however, if you can accomplish that, it makes the rest of the process so much easier! Some people ask friends and family who they see; some use Google to find providers and read reviews left by patients; some try several providers until they find a good fit. Some do all of the above.

Every clinic has different requirements for new patients. It is good to ask what you will need to get registered when you make your appointment. When a new patient visits my office, I ask them what brings them in to see me. It's open-ended, and gives my patients a chance to chat with me. I'll then ask all of the standard new patient questions. Once this is completed, I circle back to their goals. HRT is going to be different for each patient depending on goals, mental well-being, living situation and other considerations. The first visit is mostly about getting comfortable with me, getting a general checkup and forming a plan. Those are your three major goals with any new provider.

Sydni: So, if a patient comes in and they're ready to start their HRT journey, aside from general lab work, some providers may begin HRT treatment right away, while others may require additional visits? Is that correct?

Kellee: There are no real guidelines for prescribing HRT. No matter how open minded and accepting a provider is, they still may not feel comfortable or know how to prescribe HRT. Those providers are likely to refer you to an endocrinologist. The University of Louisville has a gender affirming endocrinology department and they take all insurance, including Medicaid. I have been doing research on prescribing HRT and I'm willing to start patients on HRT if we don't identify any health risks. It is important to remember it is a process. If you have the expectation that you are going to get prescribed hormones on your first visit and then that doesn't happen, you may feel defeated. Don't lose hope!

Sydni: That's really good advice. Every provider has their own way of doing things. What medications could a trans femme person expect to discuss with their provider? Are there any treatments you find are often the best combination?

Kellee: Someone looking to use estrogen to transition will need testosterone blockers and estrogen. There are two different T-blockers: Progesterone and Spironolactone. I prefer Spironolactone purely because I'm more familiar with it. But as far as I can tell from the research, both are effective. Most trans women also end up on some form of antidepressants or mood stabilizer. Let's be real, though- that is not unique to the trans community. We all need a little help these days. It is really up to me to offer my patients all of the information I have. They are driving the bus. So if they have a preference and there are no contraindications, I let them choose.

Sydni: That's a really empowering way to let the patient feel involved in their care. As a provider, what changes do you want to see regarding access to affirming care for trans people?

Kellee: My hope is that we as providers will become more comfortable and empowered to prescribe gender affirming care and advocate for our patients. The coding exists already to charge insurance for the care. The National Institute of Health published HRT recommendations for patients transitioning to male or female. They aren't necessarily recognized guidelines but they are helpful. Many patients don't have insurance and cannot be referred to a specialist.

What providers don't like to admit is that things that are unfamiliar to us terrify us! Those of us that are rude and dismissive are doing so because we HATE to admit we don't know something. We don't have to know everything but it's our job to fight for our patients and what is best for them. I hope in 2023 more providers will be brave enough to admit we don't know everything. We still have a lot to learn, and we must be willing to learn. All it takes is having the conversation.

Sydni: Is there any final advice you'd like to give or words of encouragement you'd like to provide to readers?

Kellee: We didn't touch base with the transition process for trans men, but it is much the same—only they need testosterone instead of estrogen. Testosterone is a scheduled medication. So trans men should make sure their provider can prescribe controlled substances. (Note: Kellee cannot prescribe testosterone, so we kept the focus on what she's familiar with.)

I just want to say, as corny as it sounds, things do get better! There is hope! If you are feeling hopeless or lost, reach out to friends or family. If you don't have that, call the suicide prevention hotline by dialing 988 or visit your local ER and ask for help. There are wonderful providers out there. You are not alone.

I'm grateful Kellee was able to join me for this conversation, as she's been a huge asset for me in taking better care of myself, as well as to the friends I've referred to her.

Additional resources can be found at transhealthcareresources.com.

Kellee Duke: https://www.fhclouisville.org/bs/providers/ms-kellee-duke-msn-fnp-bc/

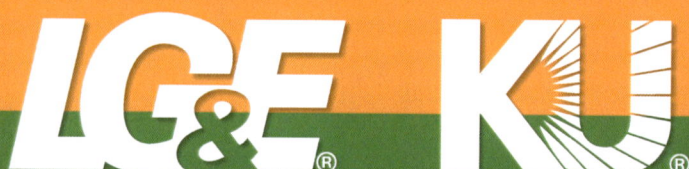

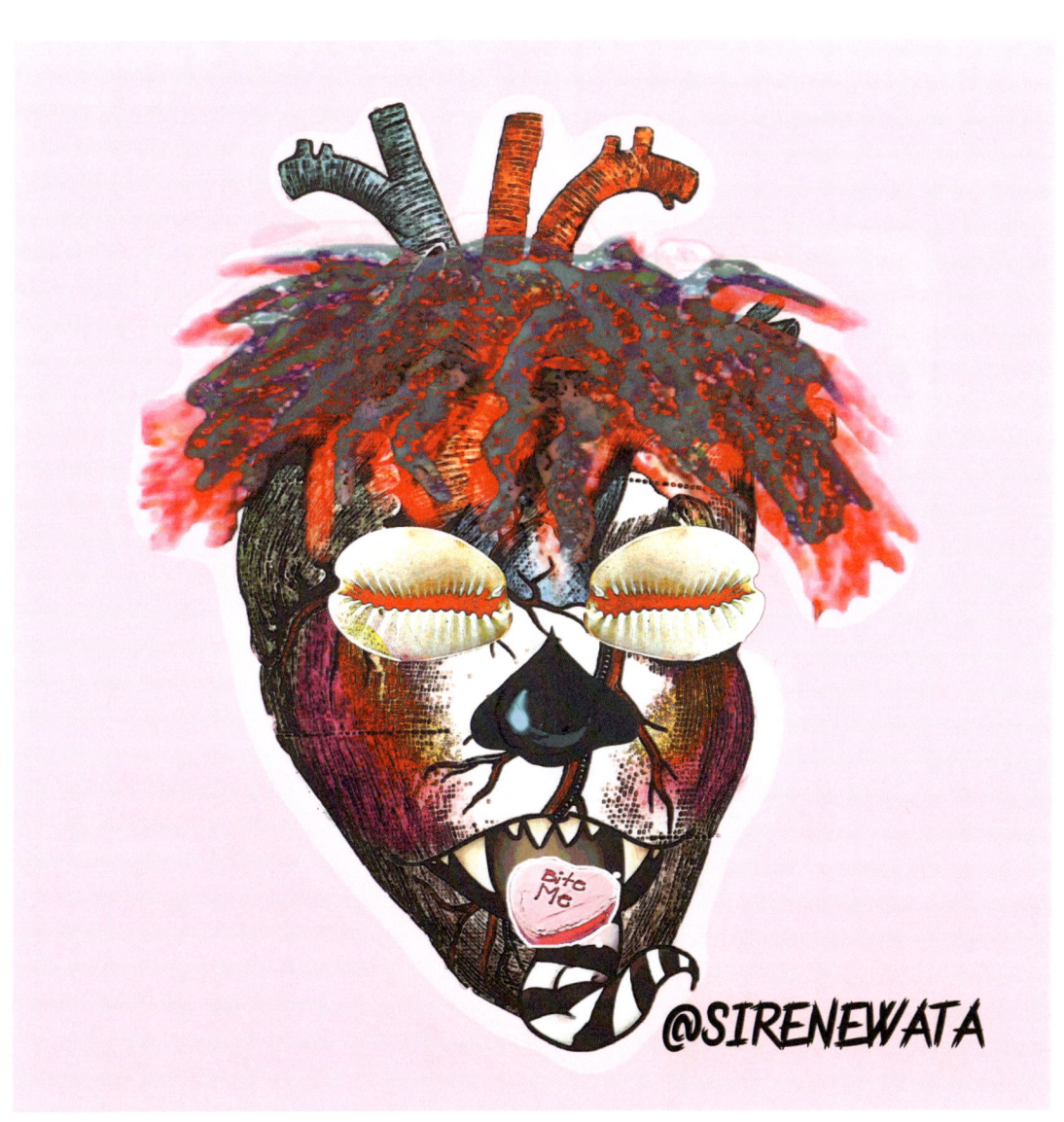

HEART CHARMER
Sirene Wata *she/they*

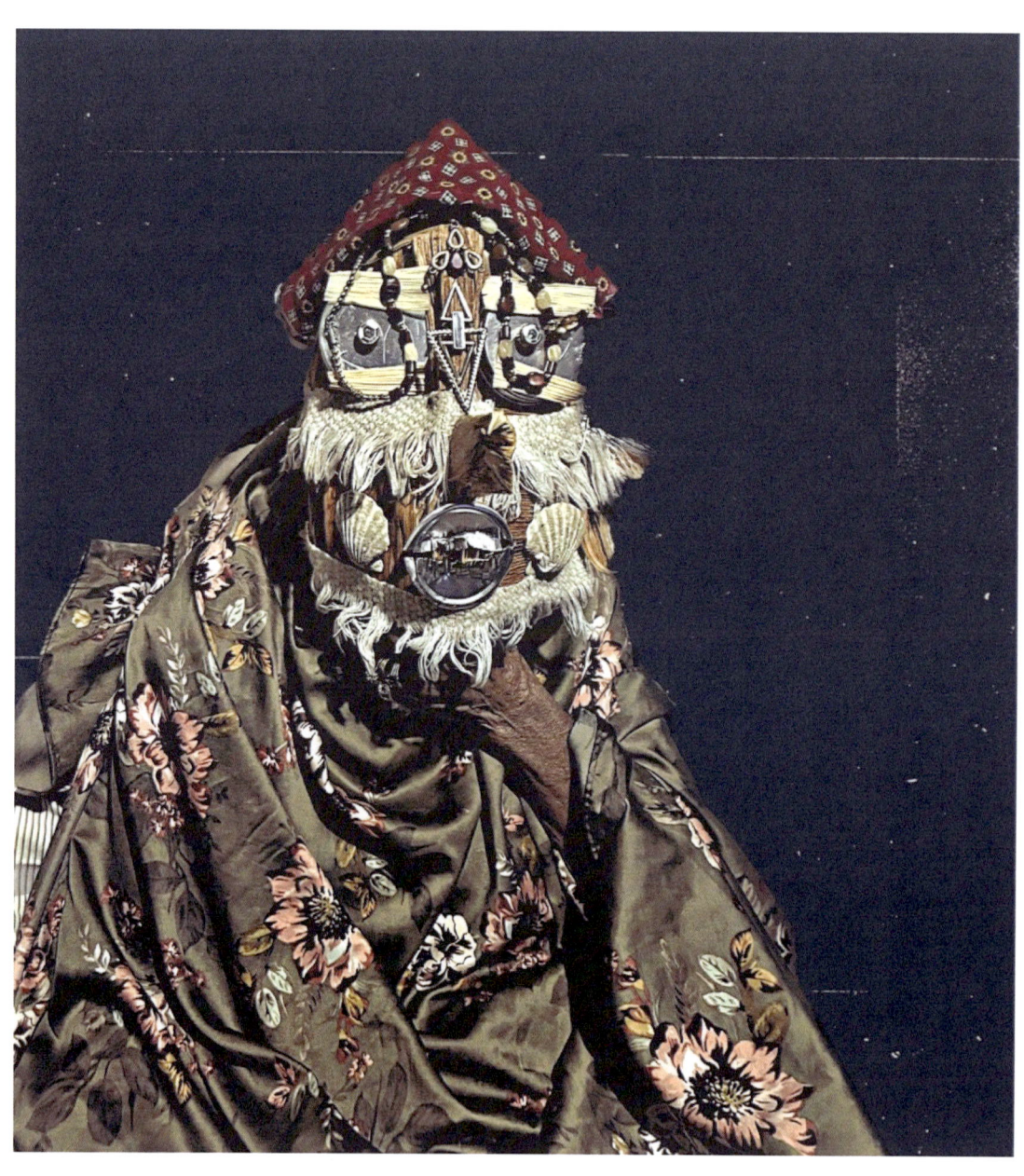

GRAN-GRAN
Sirene Wata *she/they*

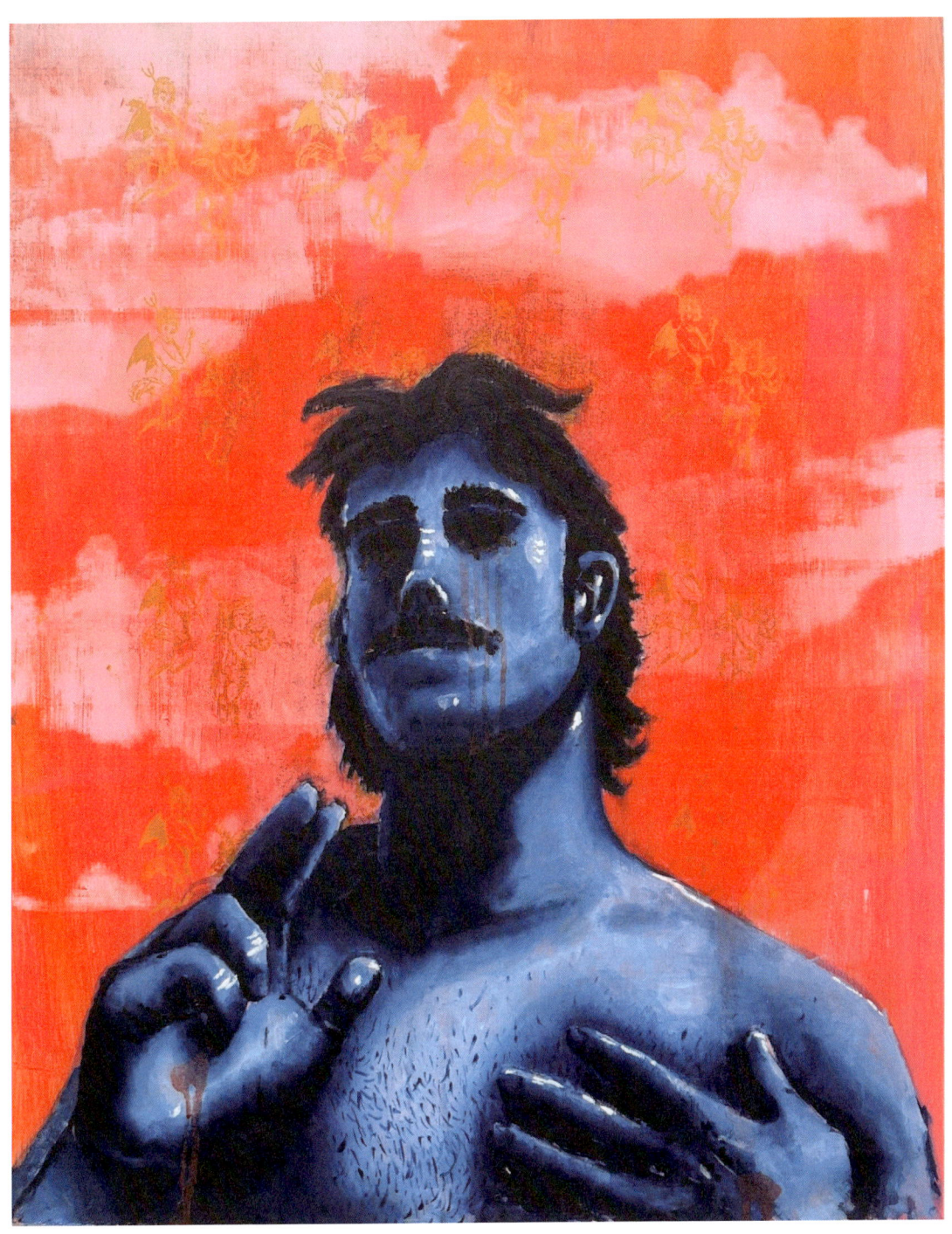

RECONCILE
Alex Blom *he/they*

Microaggressions Matter for Queer Health Justice

Heather Stewart, PHD she/they

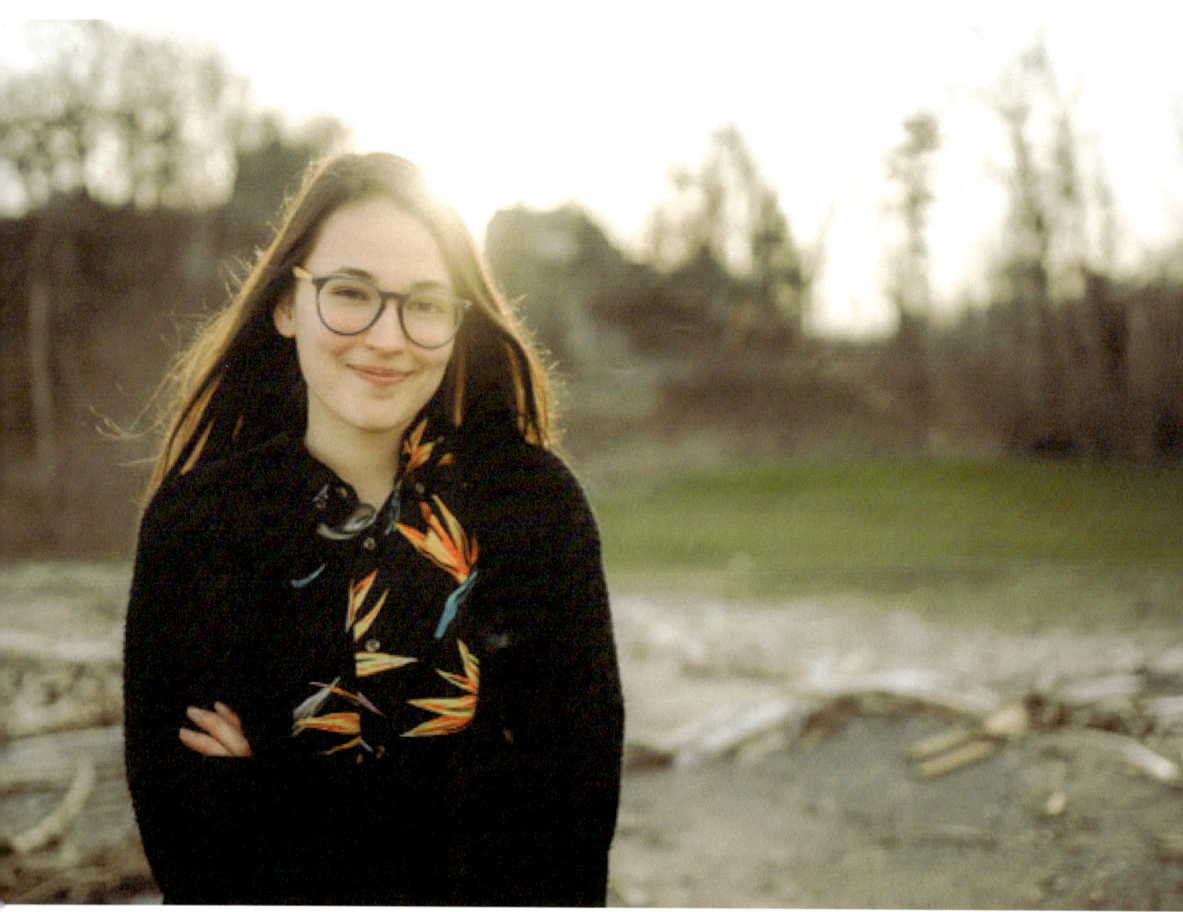

By now, the term "microaggression" is quite common and many people have a general sense of what microaggressions are – especially if they find themselves on the constant receiving end of them. Among researchers who study the phenomenon, microaggressions are typically defined as frequent and seemingly subtle insults, slights, dismissals, or snubs, which communicate bias or hostility to someone on the basis of one or more marginalized identities that they hold.

Though microaggressions can seem like minor and often unintentional "mistakes" from the perspective of those committing them, they can be deeply harmful for those who are on the constant receiving end of microaggressive comments and actions.

LGBTQ+ people are susceptible to microaggressions in all walks of life, given the persistent stigma against LGBTQ+ identities and experiences. Though microaggressions can be detrimental in any and all contexts in which they occur, they can be especially harmful when they occur in healthcare settings. This is because healthcare contexts are especially prone to power imbalances, since patients, especially patients from marginalized groups, are often in vulnerable states when seeking treatment or care. This is especially true in our current sociopolitical context, in which LGBTQ+ people are seeking health care against the backdrop of legislative attacks on their communities, identities, and their very ability to access what can be lifesaving care.

In medical contexts, microaggressions against LGBTQ+ are common, though they might go unnoticed by cisgender/heterosexual providers, staff, and patients. Consider some examples:
- Patient intake forms often exclude gender-inclusive options for sex and gender identification (thereby erasing trans, non-binary, and intersex people).
- Clinic staff and practitioners often misgender or deadname trans and non-binary patients.
- Non-heterosexual and non-monogamous people often face questions about sexual behavior that presuppose heterosexuality and monogamy.
- Medical brochures and information sheets are often written in a way that exclusively refers to binary gender identity and heterosexual sexual experience.
- Queer and trans patients are often asked irrelevant questions about their gender identities, physical bodies, or sexual behavior when those things have no bearing on the issue at hand.

These are just a few examples, though similar examples abound, and LGBTQ+ people know them all too well. Though these types of microaggressions and others often occur without malicious intent, they can cause deep harm making LGBTQ+ patients feel like they aren't being seen, heard, or understood in the ways they deserve to be. And this is important, because feeling as if one is being listened to, understood, and respected are all necessary conditions for the kinds of trust, openness, and communication that quality healthcare requires. Without these conditions, LGBTQ+ people can be further pushed out of healthcare spaces, and may avoid or delay seeking critically important care.

Minimizing the microaggressions that LGBTQ+ people face when interacting with healthcare institutions is imperative as a matter of health justice. LGBTQ+ people deserve to be seen and treated with respect in all settings, but especially in settings in which their health, well-being, and even lives depend on the ability to trust and be open with their providers.

So, how can healthcare clinics create spaces that foster a genuinely inclusive healthcare environment for LGBTQ+ patients beyond simply engaging in performative allyship? To do so requires fostering a genuine sense of belonging for LGTBQ+ patients – that is, a feeling of being recognized, taken seriously, and respected by all people in the clinical space. Here are some tips for doing so:
- Soliciting names and pronouns on intake forms and then using them consistently
- Identifying one's own pronouns (e.g., having them on staff and provider name badges)
- Having inclusive language and imagery on medical information sheets, pamphlets, and posters
- Avoiding unnecessary and invasive questioning when it is not directly relevant (and when it is relevant, using care to ensure that these issues are approached with due sensitivity)
- Soliciting input from local queer health advocates about how to be more inclusive (and compensating such advocates for their time and expertise)
- Advocating for diverse hiring practices to ensure that there is diverse representation among clinic staff at all levels
- Advocating for LGBTQ+ patients beyond the clinic – showing up for LGBTQ+ people and communities socially and politically, and being aware of how structural inequalities influence health outcomes

Though these tips are not perfect, nor are they complete, they offer an important starting place. Those who are tasked with the responsibility of providing care to anyone, and especially to the people and communities society already renders vulnerable in far too many ways, must take every step possible to avoid any preventable harm, and to promote justice at any and all costs.

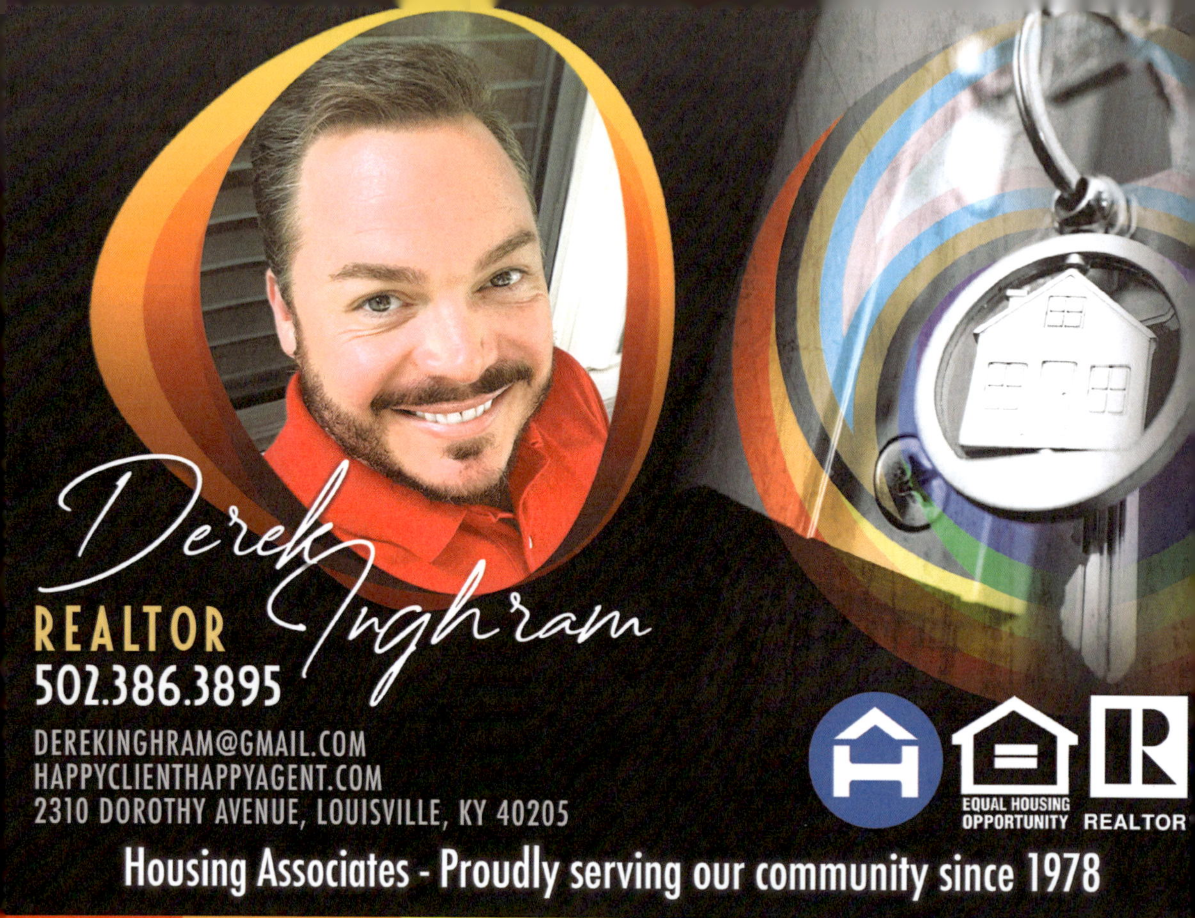

Derek Inghram
REALTOR
502.386.3895
DEREKINGHRAM@GMAIL.COM
HAPPYCLIENTHAPPYAGENT.COM
2310 DOROTHY AVENUE, LOUISVILLE, KY 40205
EQUAL HOUSING OPPORTUNITY
REALTOR
Housing Associates - Proudly serving our community since 1978

CUSTOM LogoWare
Certified LGBT
YOUR DESIGN HERE
Custom Apparel & Branded Promotional Items
www.CustomLogoWare.com

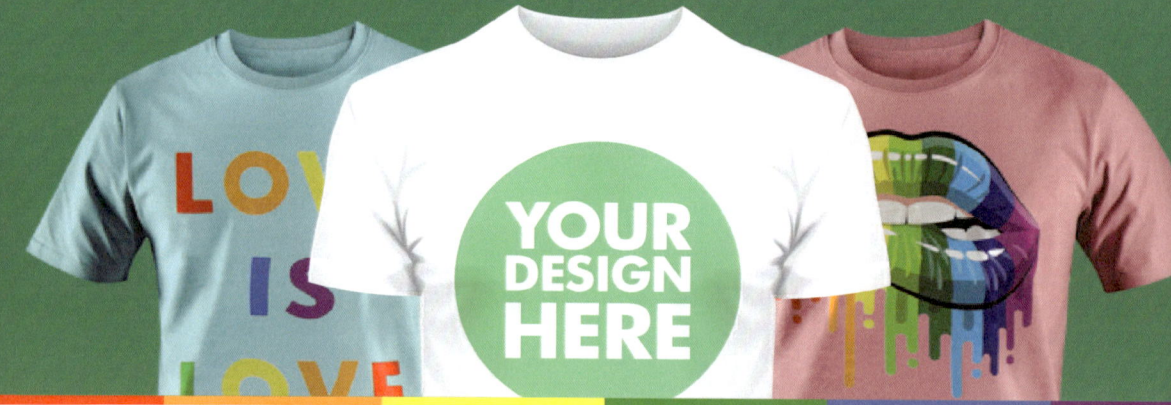

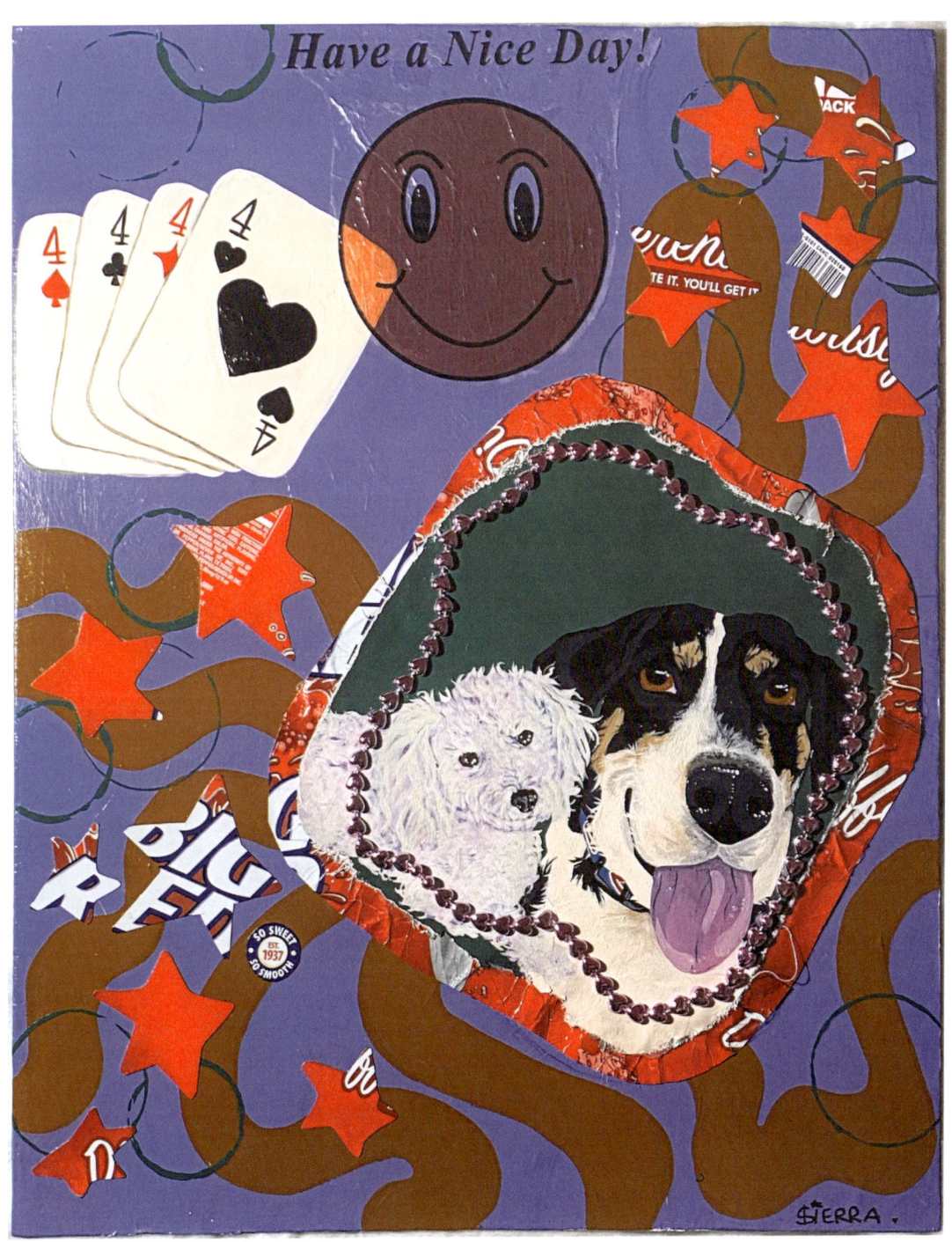

4 OF HEARTS
Sierra Durbin *they/them*

HIV Outbreak in Kentucky

Ben Gierhart he/him
Spencer Jenkins contributed to this article

We're running on three years after the height of the coronavirus pandemic, and Louisville Metro is still experiencing the consequences of the isolation and collective trauma resulting from the virus. Society has been cycling through anxiety, apathy, and grief for so long, and it has led to an historical rise in the transmission of new HIV cases, particularly in people who inject drugs (PWID).

Kentucky has had at least 54 counties that have been at a high risk for an HIV epidemic or Hepatitis C outbreak among PWID since 2016, according to information from the Centers for Disease Control and Prevention. That's nearly half of Kentucky's counties – and several of them are in the top 10 of the 220 vulnerable counties listed across the country.

In 2020, there were at least 7,911 people living with HIV in Kentucky, and there were 300 new cases of the virus diagnosed. As of January 2022, there were at least 9,200 Kentuckians living with HIV, and 340 new infections occurred.

Artwork by Andy Mendoza she/her/ella

"In Jefferson County, we have seen the highest rate of transmission for new HIV cases that we've ever seen in recorded history of the AIDS epidemic," says Michael Kopp, the founder of Social Practice Lab, a nonprofit that distributes HIV self-testing kits. Although Kopp works with the Louisville Metro Public Health and Wellness Department, the group is not involved with distributing the self-test kits.

Kopp has some ideas about why that might be.

> "I think... two things are fueling this transmission that we're seeing right now," says Kopp. "One is the Coronavirus pandemic. When this first came about, a lot of our services shut down for a while. We weren't testing people because of the social distancing measures. Other resources and people were pulled from our team to assist in the COVID response."

All social programs offer under the pressure of finite resources and harm reduction services programs especially so. It stands to reason then that a sudden depletion and/or reallocation of those resources could result in exacerbated conditions.

Kopp believes that while his program's services had reduced availability, the game has changed substantially, featuring new drugs on the scene many times more powerful than heroin. "I think that [the second contributing factor to the rising numbers are] the physiological effects of the drugs on the street now, namely fentanyl and carfentanyl. It's a way more intense high. The half-life of the high is like thirty minutes and then there's an intense urge or need to inject again because of withdrawal symptoms. So people are using more frequently and using at a higher [quantity]."

Kopp goes on to say that resources are not out there at the level they were before the pandemic and certainly not at the level they need to be with these new, unsettling trends in the community.

"People are left in isolation. A lot of people relapsed and had to come back into the program. A lot of these things are working together to create this perfect storm of what we're seeing right now in the HIV rates in Jefferson County."

It's also worth mentioning that this phenomenon is not unique to Louisville.

"[It's] statewide. I would say nationwide as well. We have community partners in Michigan that we converse with and discuss harm reduction trends and practices, and they're seeing a severe increase in transmission as well," he said.

While Kopp doesn't believe that there is a one-size-fits-all solution that will work for every community facing these troubling times, he is of the belief that it is time to think outside the box.

> "More specifically we need to increase access to testing," he said.

Kopp's mission is aligned with harm reduction, a practice that aims to mitigate the consequences of drug use. At its core, harm reduction is about practicality. It is about facing the inevitability of drug use and resultant disease transmission and developing compassionate strategies to help communities cope. Those strategies often involve education and testing, of course, but the pillars of programs such as Kopp's also go deeper: referral to social, mental health, and other medical services as well as prophylaxis — that is, specific action taken to prevent disease, in this case, HIV and Hepatitis C transmission— through abscess/wound care and syringe exchange.

The Social Practice Lab received grant funding for a program called Zeroing In - Ending the HIV Epidemic from Gilead Sciences. With that funding, Kopp and the nonprofit's partners have distributed 161 test kits for free to primarily low-income residents of Louisville since December 2022. They

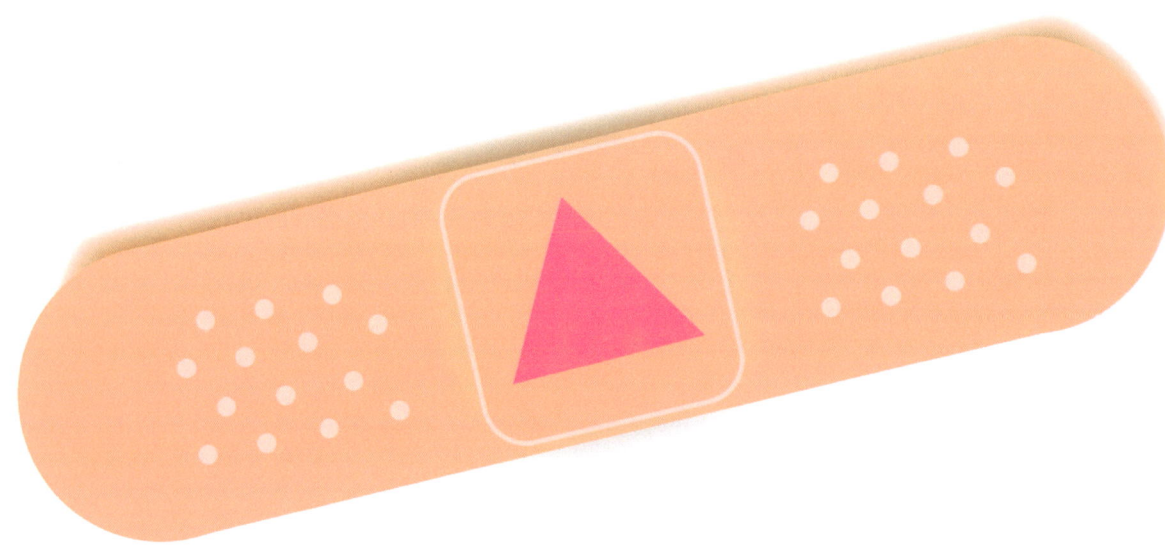

plan to wrap up distribution in the summer of 2023, Kopp said. Although the group focuses on low-income PWID, Kopp said he would "morally" have a hard time turning away anyone who asked for a self-test kit.

"This is, at its heart, an equity issue, and it's our low-income, socially and economically disadvantaged communities that are most negatively impacted by all this," he added.

The Social Practice Lab also offers folks confirmatory testing on site. Recipients of the nonprofit's self-test kits aren't required to report results, but if an initial test comes up positive, Kopp said that they can offer people a test that will confirm a positive HIV result to properly diagnose someone with HIV, Kopp said.

Louisville Public Health doesn't participate in the distribution of self-testing kits, Kopp said, but the group's Harm Reduction Outreach Services (a syringe exchange program) operates under the same roof at the Shelby Street location.

In the past, the testing had been largely stationary, on site in the health department.

Kopp has also worked hard to team up with organizations such as Feed Louisville who provide hot meals to the homeless community once a week, thus increasing his program's presence for those who require its services.

Kopp said providing the opportunity for people to self-test for HIV provides "autonomy and agency" over the individual's health. It's not an option for everyone, but for those who have had bad experiences with health care providers or those who aren't comfortable going through the testing process with a stranger, self-testing can provide an alternative to the negative experiences caused by stigma surrounding the virus.

Since the inception of the pandemic, it seems that the world changes every day, hour to hour even. With people like Michael Kopp and the rest of his team at Louisville Metro's harm reduction services program, the future may not seem any less uncertain, but it is nonetheless comforting to know that there are institutions out there still working hard to adapt and do as much good as possible.

To learn more, check out the Social Practice Lab's Medical Harm Reduction Toolkit and listen to QueerKentucky's Beards and Lavender podcast episode on the subject.

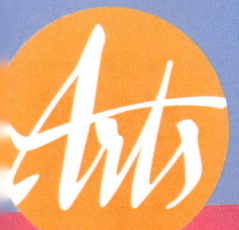

Celebrate Art in Kentucky

Support Fund for the Arts today.

FundForTheArts.Org/Give
Your gift keeps Kentucky dancing.

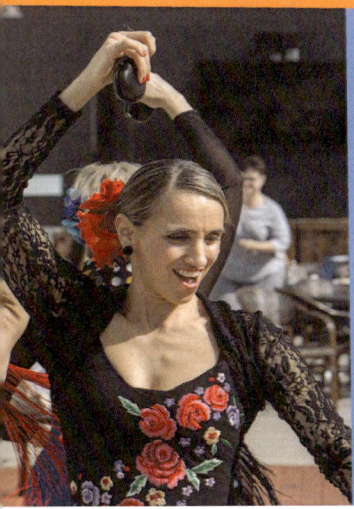
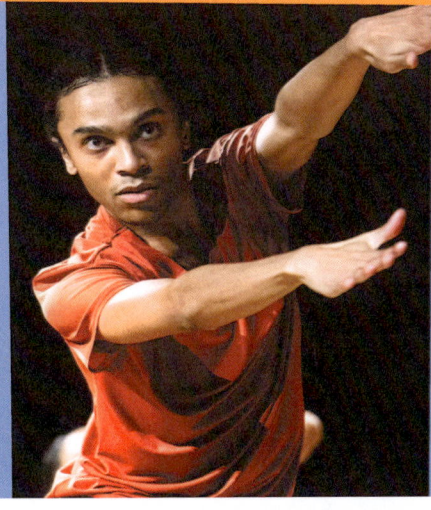
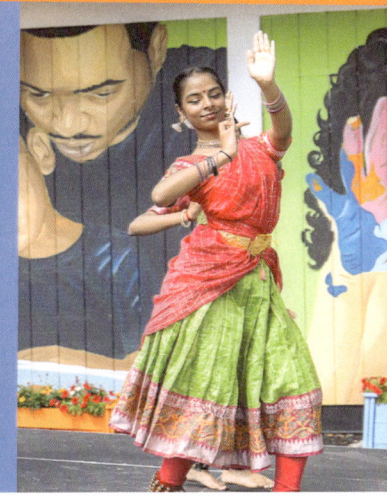

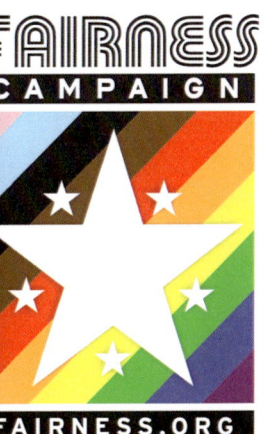

JOIN THE FIGHT FOR LGBTQ RIGHTS IN KY!

Message Your State Lawmakers **Now**!
Fairness.org/Reps

1/3 of participants were refused treatment due to their perceived gender and/or sexual identity from healthcare providers.

Based on a study conducted by UofL and KHJN,

To learn ore or for help navigating new legislation, visit
www.kentuckyhealthjusticenetwork.org

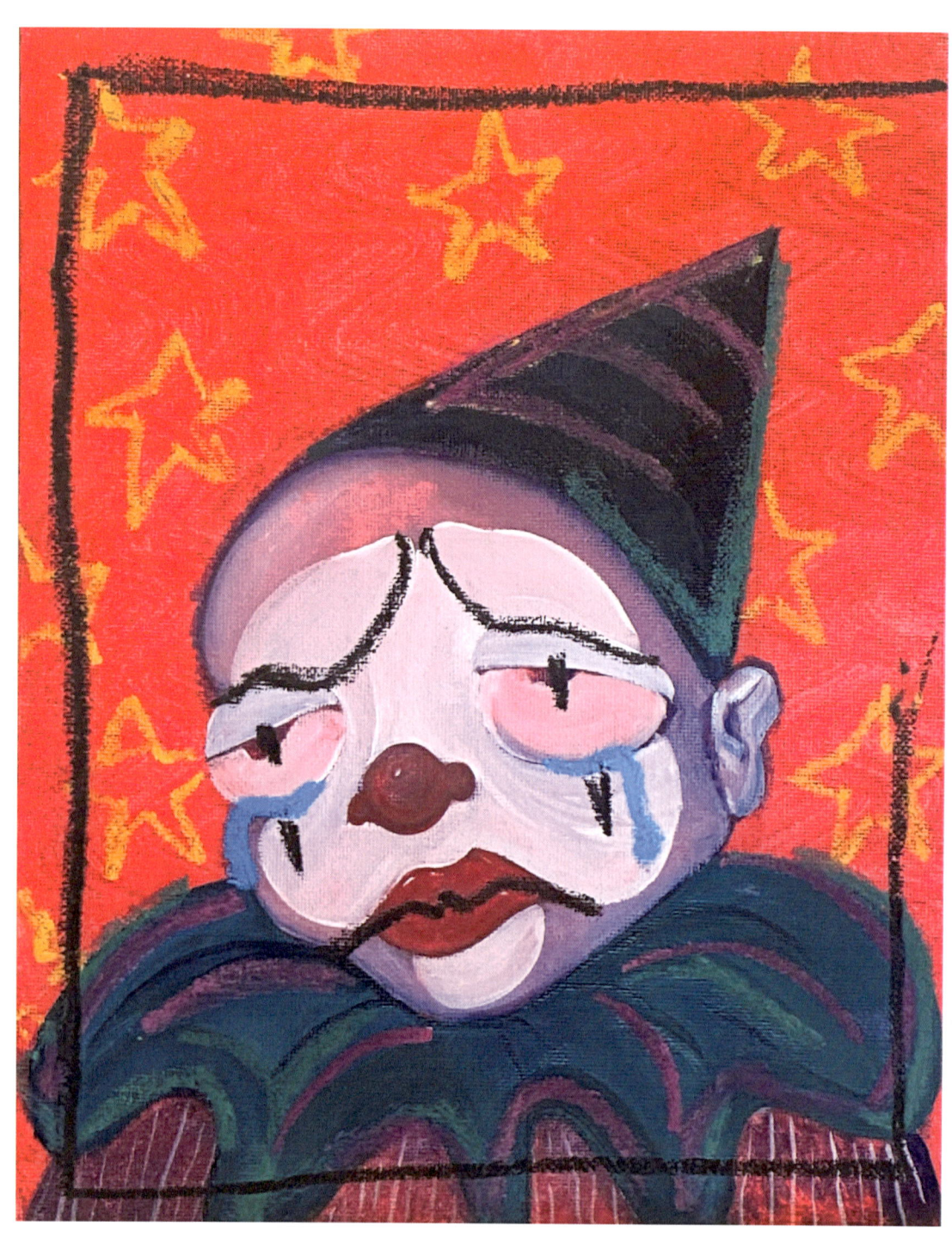

THE MASK
Sierra Durbin *they/them*

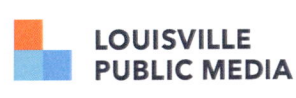

COVERING & DISCOVERING THE CITY THAT MADE US.

THE NEW LPM.ORG

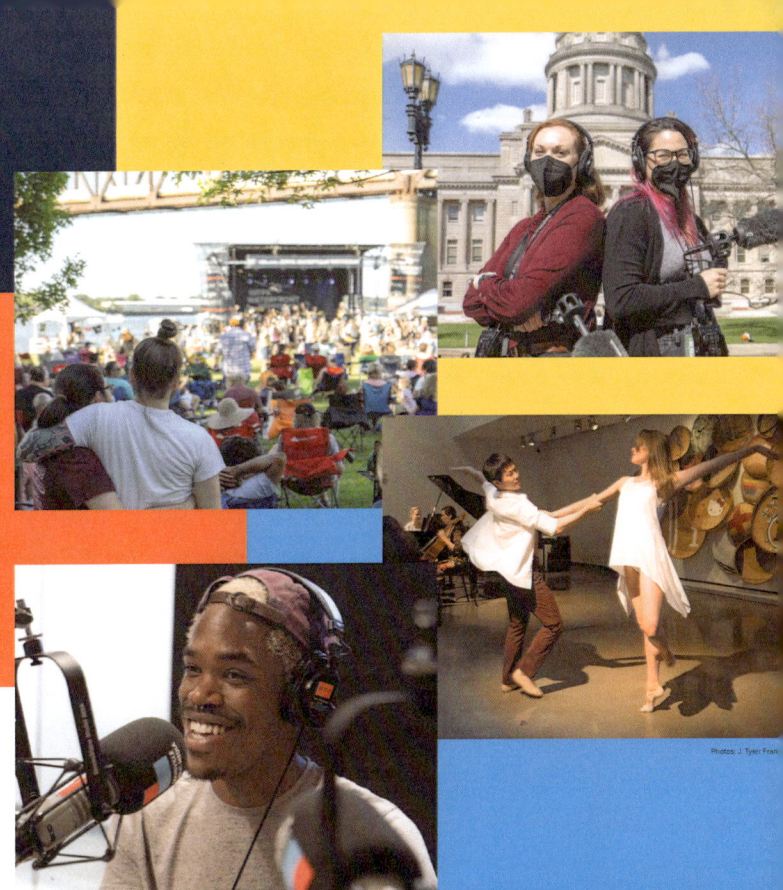

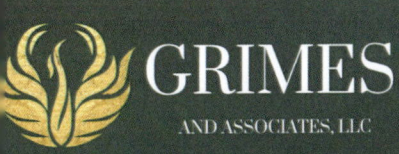
GRIMES
AND ASSOCIATES, LLC

We love working with **Dreamers**, even if you use a different word for dreams.

Bookkeeping | Financial Consulting | Payroll | Tax Planning

grimesandassociatesllc.com

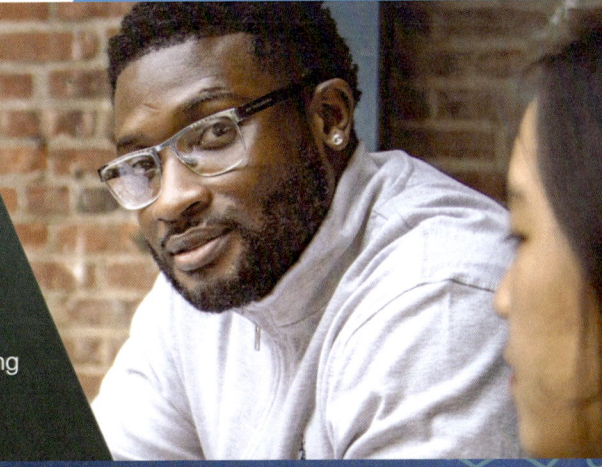

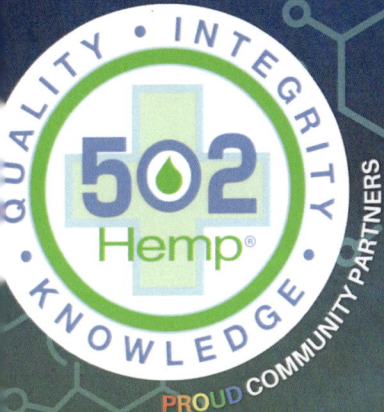

QUALITY · INTEGRITY · KNOWLEDGE
502 Hemp®
PROUD COMMUNITY PARTNERS

Your choice for
DISPENSARY GRADE
CBD products

Check us out!

Alix Thomason
she/they

Another Sexy Sex Ed Update

Artwork by Andy Mendoza   *she/her/ella*

Sexy Sex Ed is an organization for and by young people that is bringing comprehensive, evidence-based, and queer affirming sexual health education to rural Appalachia. Created by Tanya Turner, the organization began in 2012 as a workshop series for Stay Together Appalachia Youth Project, but soon requests began pouring in from all over.

Spanning over five states, the programs teach everything from sexual safety/anatomy to consent, filling in the information where most schools leave off. They now continue those workshops in places like classrooms, churches, community centers, and even parks. They also have sex ed event booths at concerts, bards, parades, and anywhere else there might be people eager to learn. Using art, dialogue, and other creative media, Sexy Sex Ed meets people of all ages where they are.

The educators come from all walks of life, from social workers and teachers to artists and students. They have also created a sexual health resource map, giving people access to book trainings, along with educator bios.

There are a lot of factors that prevent people in this area from getting the scientifically-based sex education they deserve. From politics to religion, there are many sources that try to control information and how people view their own autonomy. Even though the programming is age-appropriate and uses fact-based educational courses, Sexy Sex Ed was the target of hundreds of online threats after a popular right-wing Twitter user released misinformation about the virtual Sexy Summer Camp workshop series.

Despite this attack, the educators refuse to back down. According to their website, "Sexy Sex Ed's work providing access to comprehensive sexual education is deeply rooted in principles of political and personal consent, safety, and bodily autonomy. We teach people about their bodies, that their bodies are their own, and that all people deserve to decide what happens to their bodies without external influence or coercion. We know our work will be distorted by those with their own political agendas, but we will not be silenced. Our work is a response to the needs of the communities in which we live. It is important and essential."

Cate and Ondine, two of the educators with Sexy Sex Ed, said working in sexual education in the Bible Belt really has its own set of challenges.

"I think a lot of it is religion and the use of religion in the area. Even if people don't go to church or their family doesn't practice regularly, they still feel restricted by it…and the news," Cate said.

"There is a lot of hysteria right now, making people afraid of something that's not really there. They lie about what's actually happening."

In the Bible Belt, there is often backlash for progressive ideology. Whether it is being a part of the LGBTQIA+ community, or claiming your own bodily autonomy loudly and passionately, deeply held religious and conservative culture in the region creates barriers to engaging in progressive and justice-oriented efforts. According to Ondine, that is a big part of the issues Sexy Sex Ed is facing.

"We are held hostage by conservative governments that don't want people to have autonomy. There can be fear around it, as well as homophobia and sexism," Ondine said. "We are transparent about what our goals are: empowerment, meeting people where they are, and autonomy."

Another issue is the lack of teachers and funding. There is already a lack of educators throughout the country, and even less that have been specifically trained in sexual education. Many of the sexual health training programs that teachers can go to are very expensive, and oftentimes those teachers then end up leaving this area to go to more progressive regions.

It's difficult doing this work in the political climate we have right now, and many people trying to change it for the better are being harassed. But even when things get hard, they know their work is too important to quit. Cate knew that even after the doxxing that happened to the educators in Sexy Sex Ed, they had to keep going.

"It was really hard and traumatic. You have to be as kind with yourself as you can be, because you are doing this work for a good reason. Even though all of these people in power are saying terrible things about you, (this work) is necessary for people's lives and survival. I take time to process my feelings, but if I stay out too long we won't get the message out," said Cate.

Throughout the Bible Belt, the abstinence-only approach is pushed within communities and schools.

"In my high school education, sex ed wasn't really taught," Cate said. "We talked about the reproductive systems, the fear of disease, but nothing about consent. And you can see the way it's affected our culture, we don't really respect people's autonomy."

But in the Sexy Sex Ed workshops, consent is woven into every part of it. It is the primary foundation of their teachings, from verbal consent to nonverbal consent, and how you can always revoke consent at any time. They want people to feel empowered around their sexuality and pleasure.

"Stigma keeps us from saying what we want and what we need," Ondine said. "There are a lot of people who are very open to it, they just aren't used to experiencing it." These classes aren't just for teens and young adults. Many older folks have never been given a proper sex education, and many of them have experienced sexual violence since they were not taught anything at all.

The South has traditionally had super low rates of contraceptive use. This is caused by pushing a shame-based sex education that is rooted in abstinence-only teachings and fear. When teenagers don't feel safe enough to talk to an adult about sex, it doesn't stop them from having it, it only stops them from learning how to do it safely.

According to the CDC, characteristics of quality sex education programs include the following:[1]

- Taught by well-qualified and highly-trained teachers and school staff
- Use strategies that are relevant and engaging for all students
- Address the health needs of all students, including the needs of lesbian, gay, bisexual, transgender, and questioning youth
- Connect students to sexual health and other health services at school or in the community

Their study on sex education says "Quality sexual health education provides students with the knowledge and skills to help them be healthy and avoid human immunodeficiency virus (HIV), sexually transmitted diseases (STD), and unintended pregnancy." It has also been shown in countless studies that access to comprehensive sex education lowers intimate partner violence, STIs, and homophobia, and transphobia.

Sexy Sex Ed is primarily funded by the Appalachian Community Fund and the Kentucky Health Justice Network, but there are lots of ways you can help too. You can donate money directly to the organization, or donate supplies such as condoms, Plan B, and gas cards. You can also follow their Facebook or Instagram page and help share the information content on social media, or even host an event.

[1] *"What Works: Sexual Health Education." Centers for Disease Control and Prevention, Centers for Disease Control and Prevention, 3 Feb. 2020, https://www.cdc.gov/healthyyouth/whatworks/what-works-sexual-health-education.htm.*

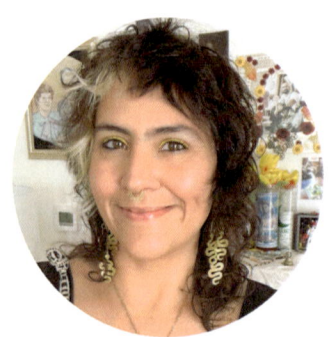

According to the CDC, characteristics of quality sex education programs include the following:

1 Taught by well-qualified and highly-trained teachers and school staff

2 Use strategies that are relevant and engaging for all students

3 Address the health needs of all students, including the needs of lesbian, gay, bisexual, transgender, and questioning youth

4 Connect students to sexual health and other health services at school or in the community

A FIGHTING CHANCE: QUEER YOUTH, EDUCATION EQUITY, AND MENTAL HEALTH

Belle Townsend
she/they

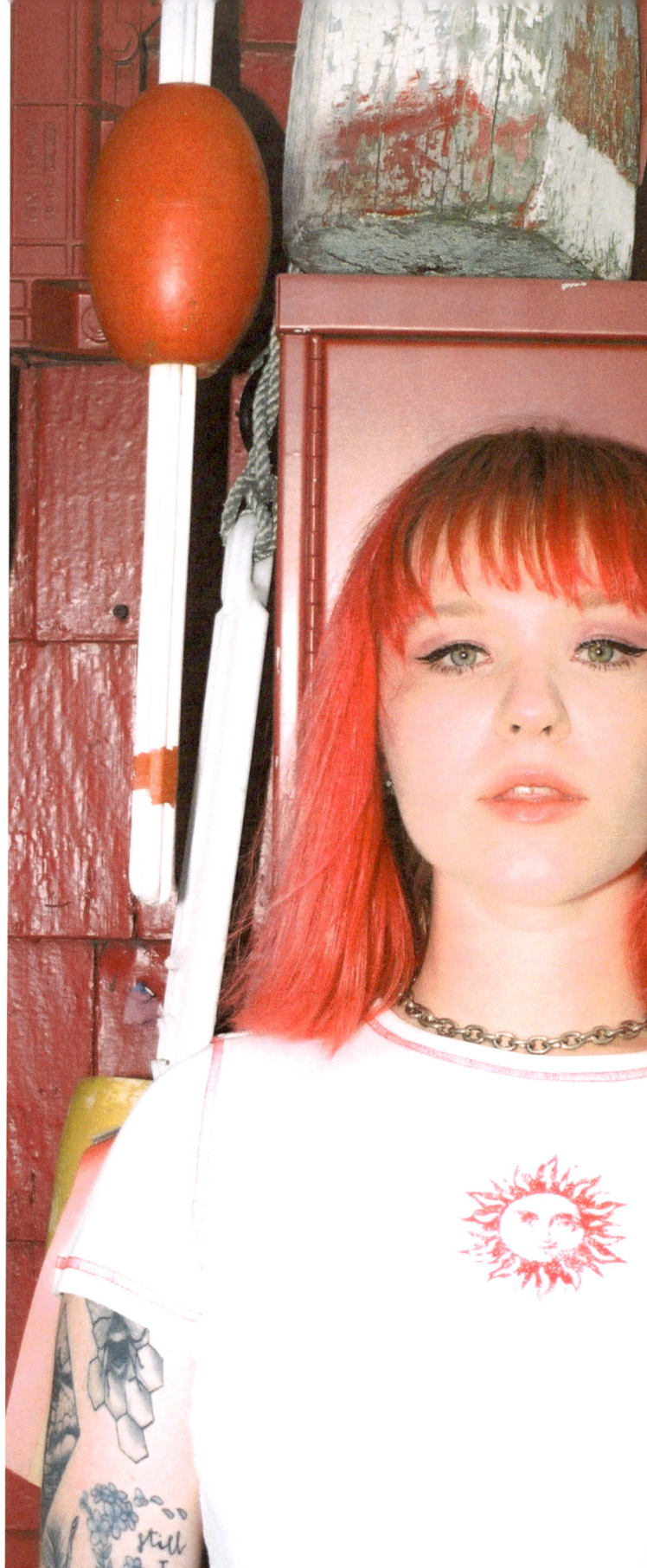

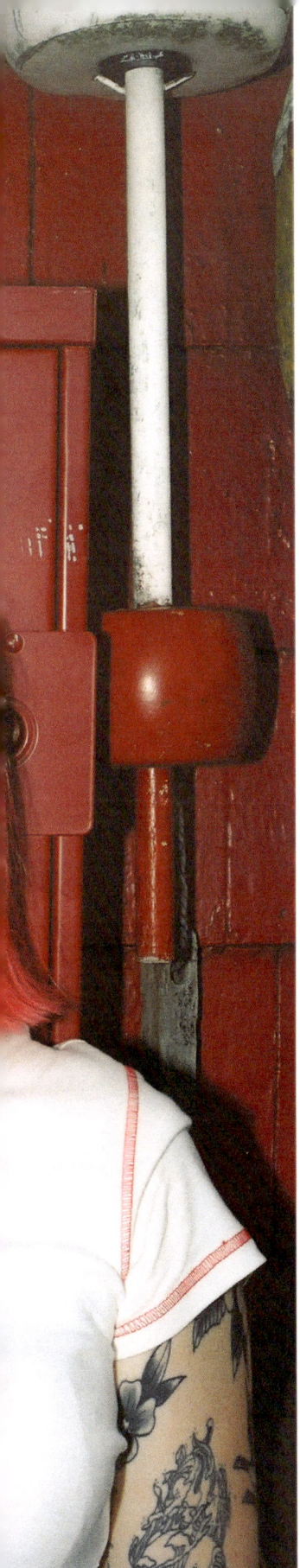

You will never hear me telling a bigot that I hope their child turns out to be queer. That is not a punishment to any good parent, given that a parent who perceives their child being queer as a punishment is creating that reality for themselves. We choose what social constructs to perpetuate. But, the only person being punished in that situation is the child forced to navigate queerness thinking that they are wrong, alone, and doomed.

There has been a nationwide push from conservative legislators to remove books and other media that provide perspectives about diverse lived experiences - or in other words, perspectives not aligned with fascist, white supremacist ideals. This has been a culminating movement for a while now, especially given the context that state-regulated curriculum has never centered on historically accurate and properly contextualized education.

This movement has been intentionally branded as "parental choice" in children's education, and not for what it actually is: erasing stories that do not fit within ideologies of white supremacy. You see, the true history and stories of lived experiences of diverse Americans cannot coexist with the false reality that capitalism and white supremacy require in order to keep functioning and marginalizing individuals.

The framed narrative is that parents deserve a right to decide on what their children learn in schools, and that there is a liberal indoctrination being performed by state-run schools. It is imperative to label this movement for what it is – fascist and white supremacist – as well as to advocate for the Black, Indigenous, brown, queer, neurodivergent, and other marginalized students who, if this movement is successful, will no longer have access to the stories of those before them.

`The stories before us often serve as maps for how to traverse the difficult landscape of being traumatized by surviving the oppressive systems that make our lives so hard. Not having access to that history and those stories is costing people their lives.`

I know what it is to be a young, queer, autistic student, raised in a Christian, white supremacist vacuum. I know the extreme isolation, the ever-present shame, the all-consuming fear... I know it all. Without access to queer media, until I was in middle school, I had no evidence that there was nothing wrong with me. Even once I had access to that media, I struggled immensely with my mental health, self-image, and relationship with the world. This is to say that my life did not have to have as much suffering as it did, and the queer students having those stories taken away from them right now do not have to be suffering in the way that they are. Let us not forget that they are suffering right now.

America was built on the foundation of racism, white supremacy, and capitalism, which all require withholding education from the oppressed as a means of continuing to perpetuate the oppressive systems.

Misinformation was a hot-button topic during the 2016 and 2020 elections when it was widely talked about that constructed media run by corporate interest is inherently anti-democratic. But, we need to keep talking about it in a broader context. Queer people are here, taking up space, and so our stories deserve to do the same. Our best combatant is good public education that provides students with the perspectives and stories that not only make them feel okay in their lived experience, but confirm their lived experience, and also help them to keep surviving their lived experience.

There are people who want to erase us from history, as well as the present and future. They have rewritten the past time and time again. But, what they cannot do is rewrite the present. We are writing it right now. To ensure that our story is told correctly, we have to show up in local politics to support public education and access to diverse media.

People talk about mental health as if it is separate from capitalism, marginalization, circumstance, and lived experience. For many of us, and for queer youth, the answer is not in suicide prevention walks and social media posts about how people need to be better at reaching out when they feel alone.

The solution to the "mental health crisis" is in tangible social change and community support that improves the everyday lives of those who white supremacy culture has fought to erase. Further, the solution lies in ensuring that young people have access to support through narratives of the present that are not only objectively true and affirming but indicative of a world that is more bearable to survive in.

Ensuring that young people, including queer students, have access to history and stories that affirm, contextualize, and support them is a necessary step in improving the mental health of young queer people.

Belle Townsend is a poet, author, political organizer, researcher, as well as small business owner from Henderson, Kentucky. Their business is currently based in Louisville, KY, where she provides services for writing, researching, editing, consulting, and baking specialty custom cakes and cupcakes. For more about the author, their services available, or about their self-published and signed author's copies of her books, Push and Pull & The Observer Effect, please visit www.belletownsend.com.

✨ **Business support that meets you where you are!**
Inclusive and training-focused business support

Website Design | Branding Design
Graphic Design | Marketing Support

Alight Agency is Queer, Appalachian, and Woman Owned, ready to help you run your business with confidence and joy. ✨

AlightAgency.com | @AlightAgency | (859) 351-3542

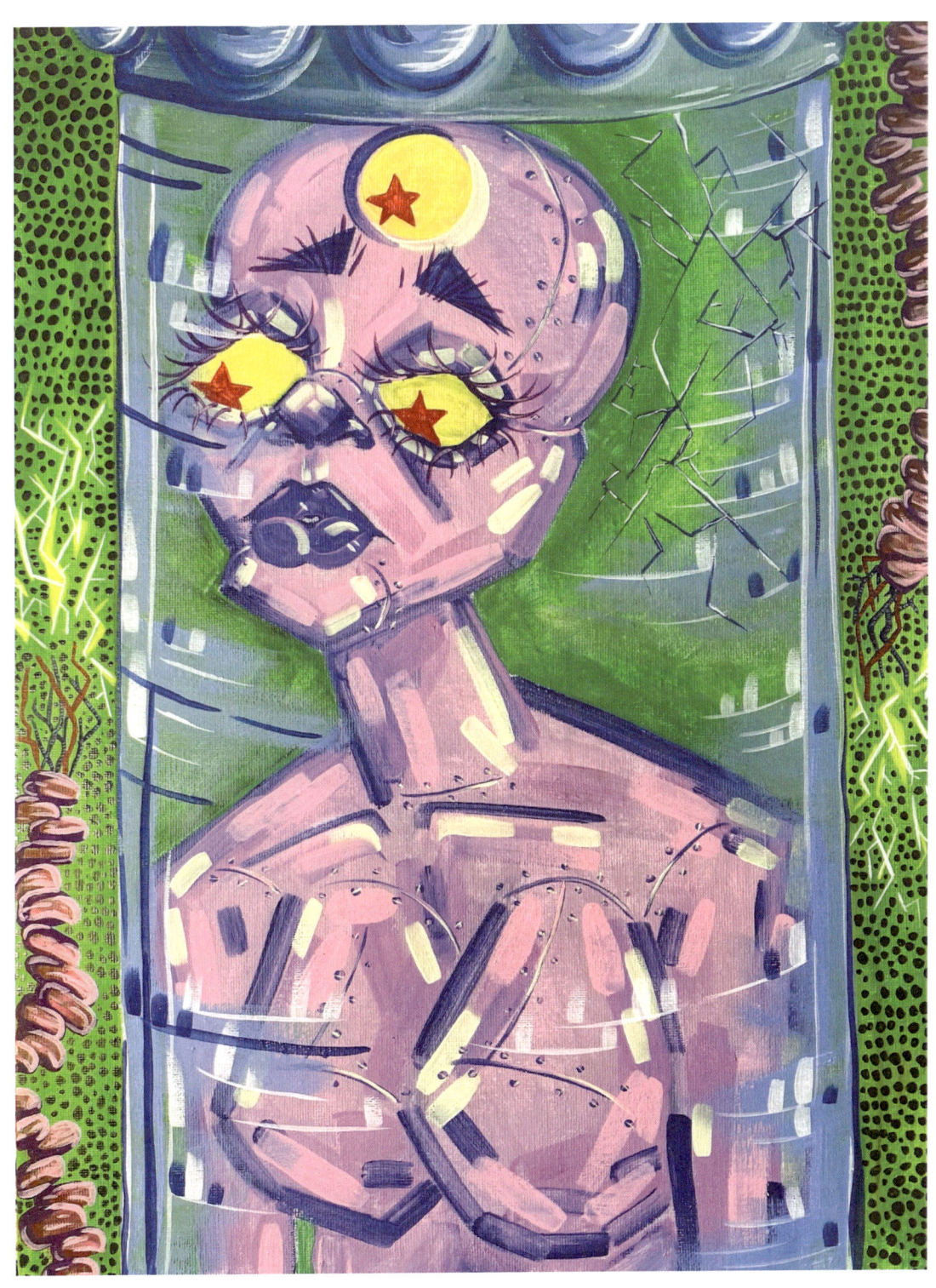

ERROR
Sierra Durbin *they/them*

Body Horror

THE QUEER AND THE MACABRE

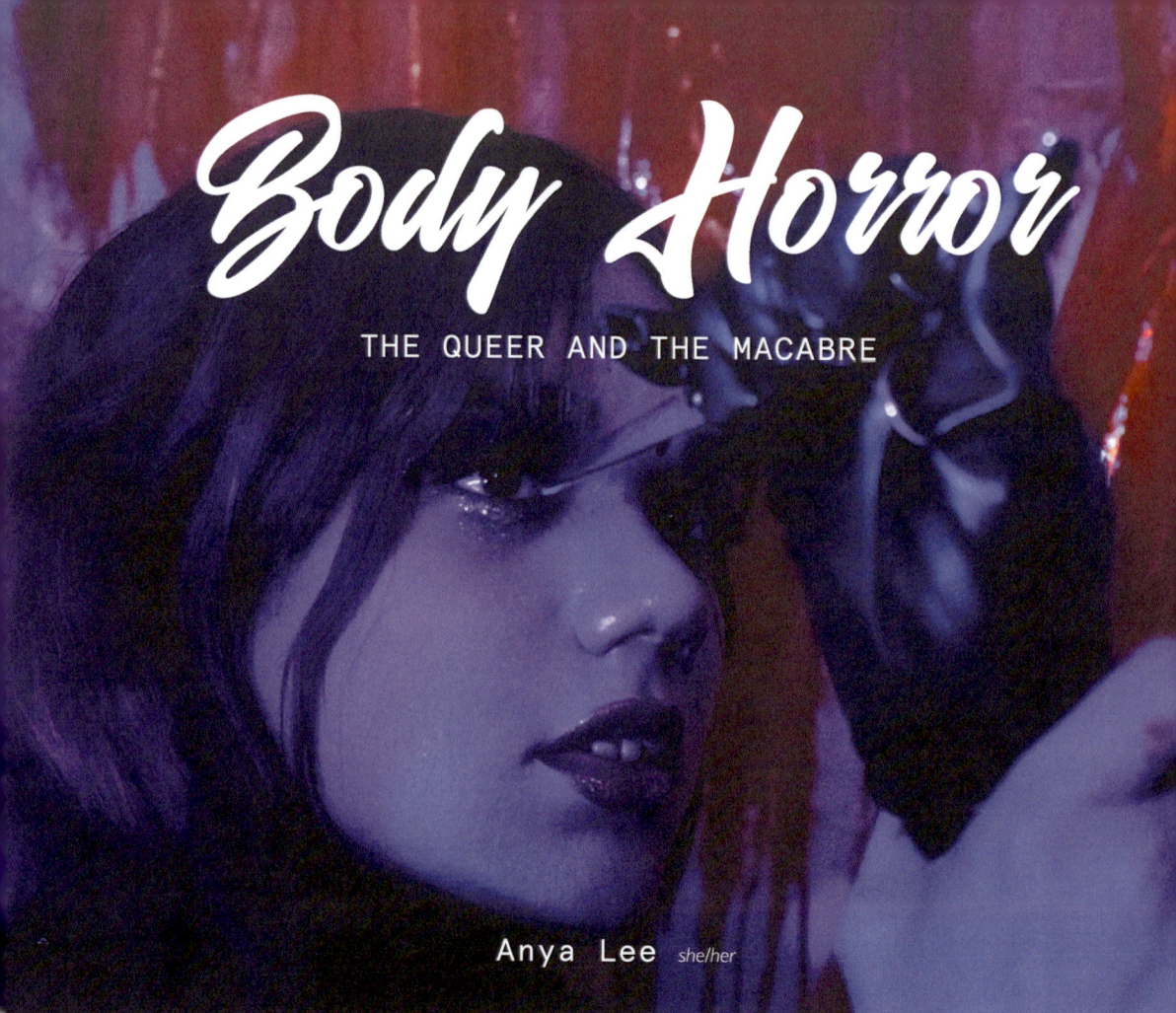

Anya Lee she/her

As one of my closest friends facetimes our transgender groupchat from post-surgery in Texas, her face is bruised, bloodied, hammered. Her face swollen into a newfound beauty, jaw shaved and skin glossy with sweat. Her eyes are swollen from lid to undereye, painted purple and black with bruising: an elegant eyeshadow that cost thousands. Her scalp sliced open with visible lines of stitching and scabbing, reattached lower to suit her new skull shape, bandaging rendering her nose, which is now slightly upturned, invisible to sight. Her head is wrapped in bandages and ice-packs like a hellish medical babushka. She smiles faintly, and we're overjoyed — she is affirmed. She is lovelier than before, achieving a goal we set out to have, too. We celebrate, we jest, we are genuinely happy for the brutal assault upon her face, because for all of the violence and mutilation that went into this product, it will melt like ice into a new incarnation of Venus, a feminine beauty she was deprived of at birth, and had to seek liberation from at the blade of a bloodied scalpel. This is joy, this horror: and this horror is so closely linked to the lives of transwomen, that this cruel desire is an intrinsic part of our reviled beings.

With a transgender actress mounting the role of Pinhead / The Priestess for the remake of Clive Barker's "Hellraiser", it wasn't exactly difficult to find vitriol online about the change in the character's portrayal, as it had already been rooted in popular iconography as having a particular look regardless of the androgynous portrayal in the novelization. But that vitriol — the adverse reactions, the spewing of unasked for opinions, the frustration of Pinhead now being a woman are all very boring, and ignore a reclamation of a problematic frontier of horror; the transwoman's place in horror, and its authenticity.

Transgender people, in the midst of our transitions, become a sort of Frankenstein's monster in full coverage foundation: to ease the woes of dysphoria and the ever present issue of being seen as something we aren't, transgender women undergo some of the most mutilating (and affirming) surgical procedures known to man, and we do so with great cost. Transition rarely ends at HRT (which transgender people are losing access to) which physically warps and alters our bodies in what could be compared to rolling a dice. You don't know the outcome, you're unaware of what changes may occur to your mood (will you become more pleasant, or emotionally terrorize your friends and family?). Your body will also distort unpleasantly: while i cannot make a truly informed opinion of the body post testosterone, I am aware that many transmen undergo hair loss, a deepening of the voice, and violent, violent acne.

But more interesting than the experimental medication we take and hormones we stuff our bodies with to incite internal change are the procedures we elect and take and save for and suffer for to be affirmed on the outside. Only in transgender circles is having your entire face sliced open, peeled off from the scalp, and laid open as a flap while blood is sucked from you with a hose and your skull is shaved down with a variety of machinery a goal. To some, this sounds like a form of torture, and to transwomen, this sounds like a form of liberation.

What is a bit of physical trauma compared to a lifetime of it otherwise? What is being cut open physically, when you contemplate doing it to yourself anyways after glancing at yourself incorrectly? Who better than a transwoman to convey a deity-like figure responsible for providing salvation through barbarism? Who else, other than a person from a group of people who routinely idolize and aspire to have their faces ripped off and bones hammered in, could properly convey this horror?

Transwomen are underutilized in horror for our experiences, but have existed in the medians of horror for a long time: the fear of cross-dressers, of deviants on the outskirts of society, the fear of the androgynous and what it presents — in horror, the stereotypes associated with trans people were misapplied, misconstrued, and taken to create paranoia and misinformation about us.

Media is rife with the portrayal of a queer coded, effeminate villain, as femininity itself is often demonized. What is more demonized, then, than a man who has become feminine? The suburban figure of terror, who threatens your masculinity with a miniskirt and wink? The fear of the unknown, the unstandard, the deviant — that with our deceptive forms and shapeshifting, we become creatures of the night that skulk around, plotting to rob men of their masculinity and patriarchal strengths is applied to us against our will, myth becoming monstrosity. And it's all very fake — It's unfounded, it's unreal. There is no cruel practice, other than what we endure for survival.

Growing up consuming violence and horrific media, the only representations of transwomen I saw were as villains, corpses, or sex workers, and usually some mix of these categories. Displayed as unambiguously the victim or a joke-induced villain, with no actual connection to any of the violence of horrors we actually endure, Clayton is a sigh of relief, an actual connection to our actual horrors.

For some transwomen, our goal is to become monsters of our own design, plotting and planning ways to achieve physical alteration, a mutation from our default states into our fantasies and the person we believed we should've been born as — and in the process, we shed tears, blood, sweat, skin, bone, fat, muscle, guts, souls. We, in some cases, participate actively in our own dehumanization to seek the life we desire as a completed person, a real human — no cost is too high for some. The mental illness, the trauma, the suffering, the marginalization, and the brutality we experience in society and at our own hands to survive in society, is the plotline to a nightmare, and as denizens of the nightmare, of course there's a deep affection for the macabre.

For transwomen, body horror is always on the grocery list, and sometimes, it doesn't get marked off. This trend in horror will hopefully continue, and whether we be victim or villain or heroine, hopefully it will contain a more than tongue-in-cheek allusion to our real horrors and connectivity with the genre. The real monstrosity of our lives is far more intense, far more scary, and far more exciting than any tired narrative free from our involvement.

Queer, Neurodivergent Entrepreneur Takes a Nonbinary Approach in Helping Autistic Community

Spencer Jenkins
he/him

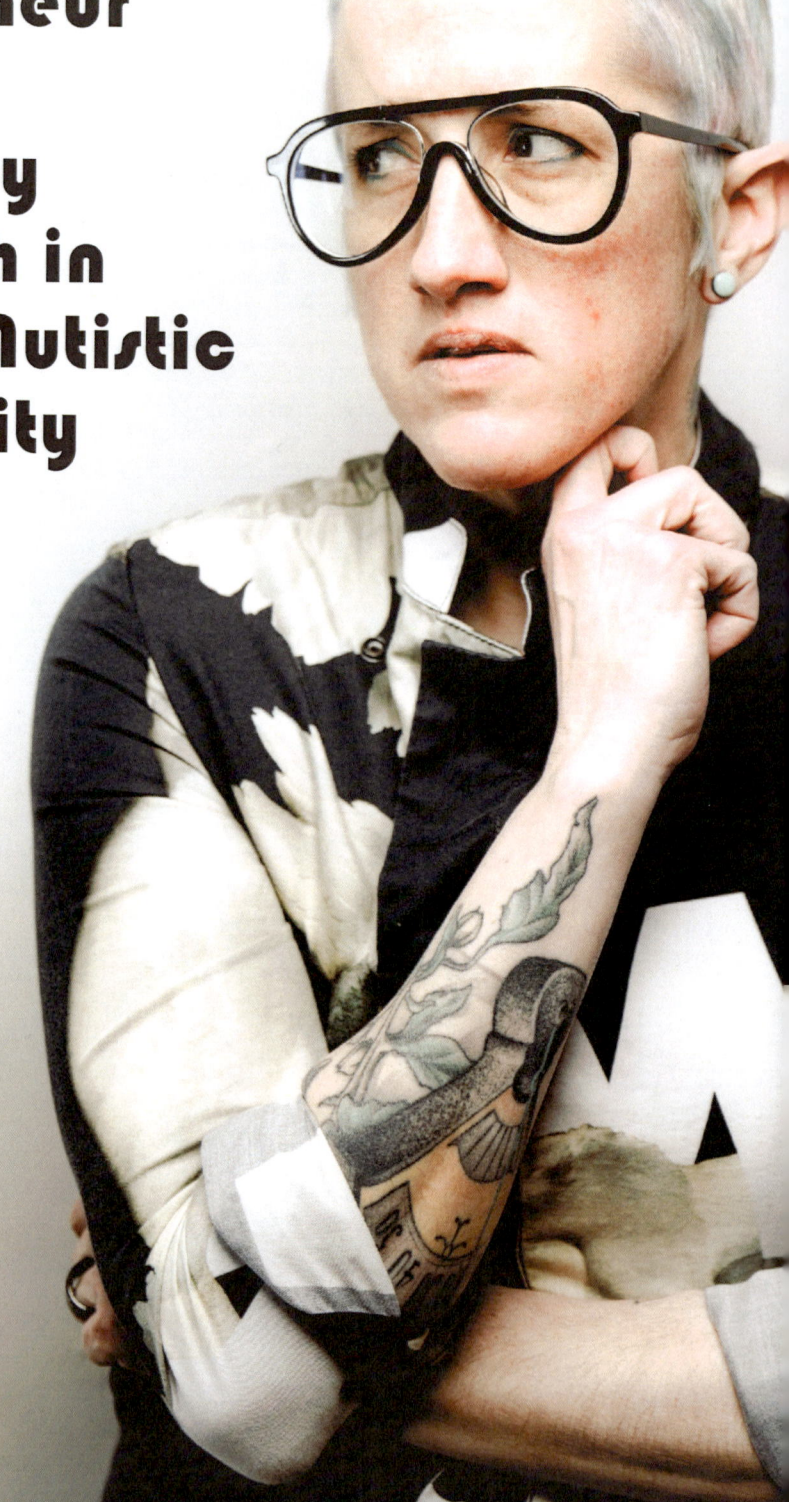

Images by Chet White   *he/him*

Kentucky's startup ecosystem comprises mainly of white, cisgender and heterosexual men.

According to StartOut, there are only TWO reported LGBTQ+ entrepreneurs in Kentucky that are considered "high-growth companies or entrepreneurs." However, every now and then, a wild card comes along and jolts the WASPy community with a delightful disturbance.

Enter Amanda Ralston, a human of many talents. A successful entrepreneur with a background in Applied Behavior Analysis (ABA). She describes herself as "charismatic, dynamic," and most notably — "compassionate." One interesting quirk? She has an unapologetic love for the Oxford comma – her one fatal flaw.

STOP, wait…ABA? Isn't that … awful?

Well, Ralston said, the early practices of ABA from the 70s and 80s included the use of punishment to create motivation to respond to certain tasks. This included water bottle sprays in the face, loud startles, and even slaps.

But, she added, just like psychology evolution, antiquated practices are abandoned in favor of more ethical and efficacious data-based practices.

"It is the simple fact that what is best practice today, will not be the same decades from now," she said. "So you must practice with humility and the ability to change with time. When you know better, you do better. But you have to have data to know better."

Many people have taken issue with the organization, Autism Speaks (known for its ABA practices), criticizing it for working to "cure" autism or viewing it as a "problem" to be "solved" (see: the puzzle piece logo of AS).

Ralston writes, "there is a very useful and needed discussion around the concept of #Neurodiversity and an always-broadening understanding that there is a wide range of needs, strengths, talents, and voices in the autism community, and beyond."

She further explains that one person with autism doesn't represent everyone with autism.

"To this point — for one group to presume to understand the preference for any family or person and the group they seek help, guidance, or affirmation from is a binary attitude. And binaries are not relevant on a spectrum."

OK, let's continue.

Being neurodivergent herself, Ralston saw a gap in the health care industry when it came to serving those with autism. To fill that need, she founded NonBinary Solutions (NBS) — an innovative decision-support software company aimed at aiding clinicians through the steps of providing care for people on the spectrum.

According to the National Autism Association, one in 44 children are on the spectrum.

Ralston is tackling the challenge of providing care to those living with autism in a unique way. By utilizing a compassionate lens and cutting-edge technology, NBS deploys interactive algorithms that guide clinicians from intake to outcome, reducing time spent on complex clinical processes.

"I have spent years listening to the needs and desires of individuals and families impacted by autism as a clinician and I've helped countless individuals learn to communicate, become more independent, safer, and happier," she said. "And a lot of that comes from experience. And a lot of experience comes from mistakes."

She adds that she's working to help other providers without her 25 years of clinical experience avoid pitfalls with supportive technology she's created.

In a February KY INNO article, Ralston said, "the software will ask providers a series of questions that correspond to internal algorithms to serve as a guide along the process, while offering the provider a list of reference materials (articles, websites) and other recommendations to help better inform decisions, while providing insurance companies a report that documents their entire work with a particular patient — and the decisions they made to reach their treatment plan."

The award-winning entrepreneur's interest in ABA began when she saw its potential to improve lives. "Autism is multidimensional, as are the people diagnosed with autism," she said. "ABA is not a one-size fits all approach. And so the solutions cannot be black and white - there must be shades of gray. Thus the name - NonBinary Solutions."

According to the Behavior Analyst Certification Board, a nonprofit corporation that was established in 1998 to meet professional certification needs identified by behavior analysts, governments, and consumers of behavior-analytic services, the number of individuals being diagnosed with autism has risen significantly over the past decade (1 in 44 people), leading to a 500% increase in the number of service providers specializing in autism.

"Having more providers is great," Ralston said. "It's important to note, however, that more than half of all service providers have less than five years of experience."

More experienced professionals are needed to help individuals with autism develop social skills, communication skills, self-care skills, and other necessary daily living skills. Additionally,

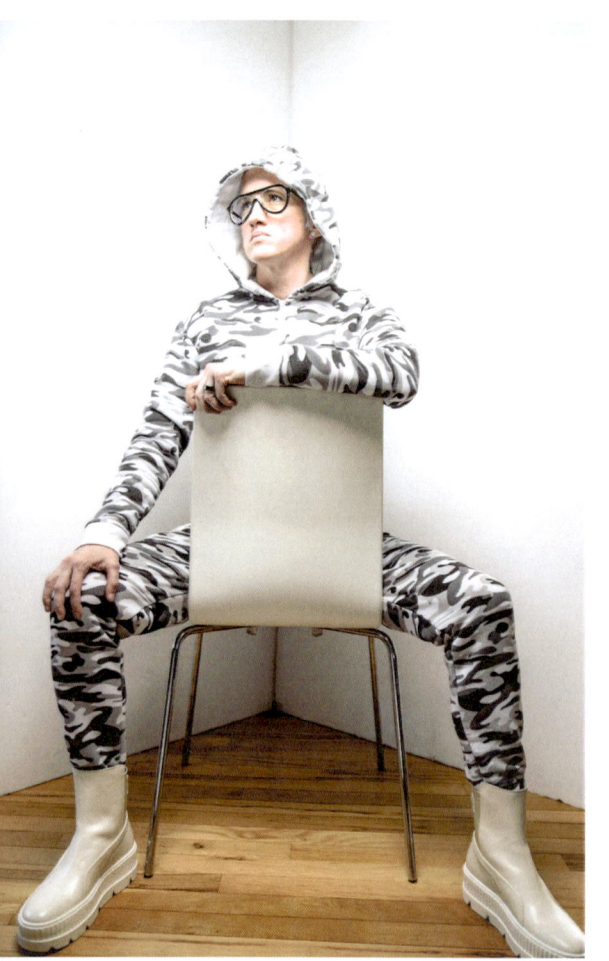
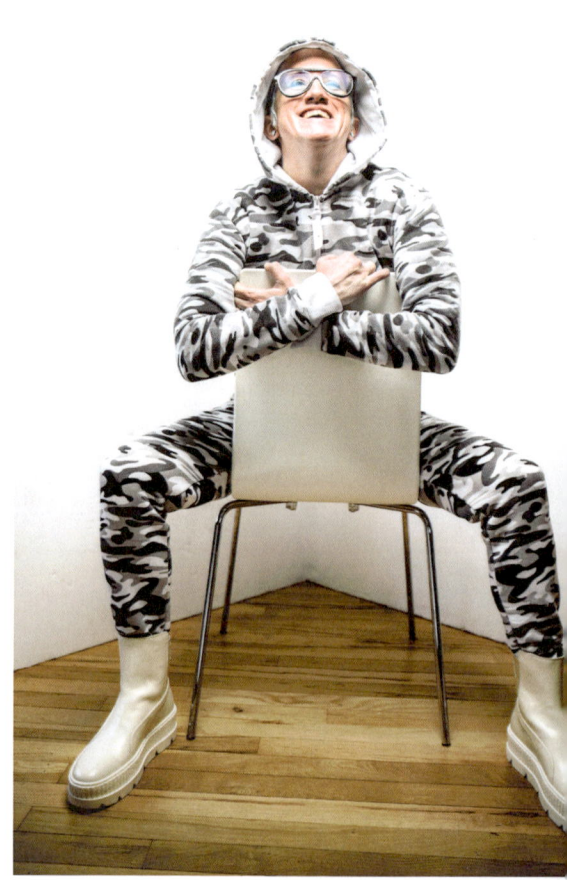

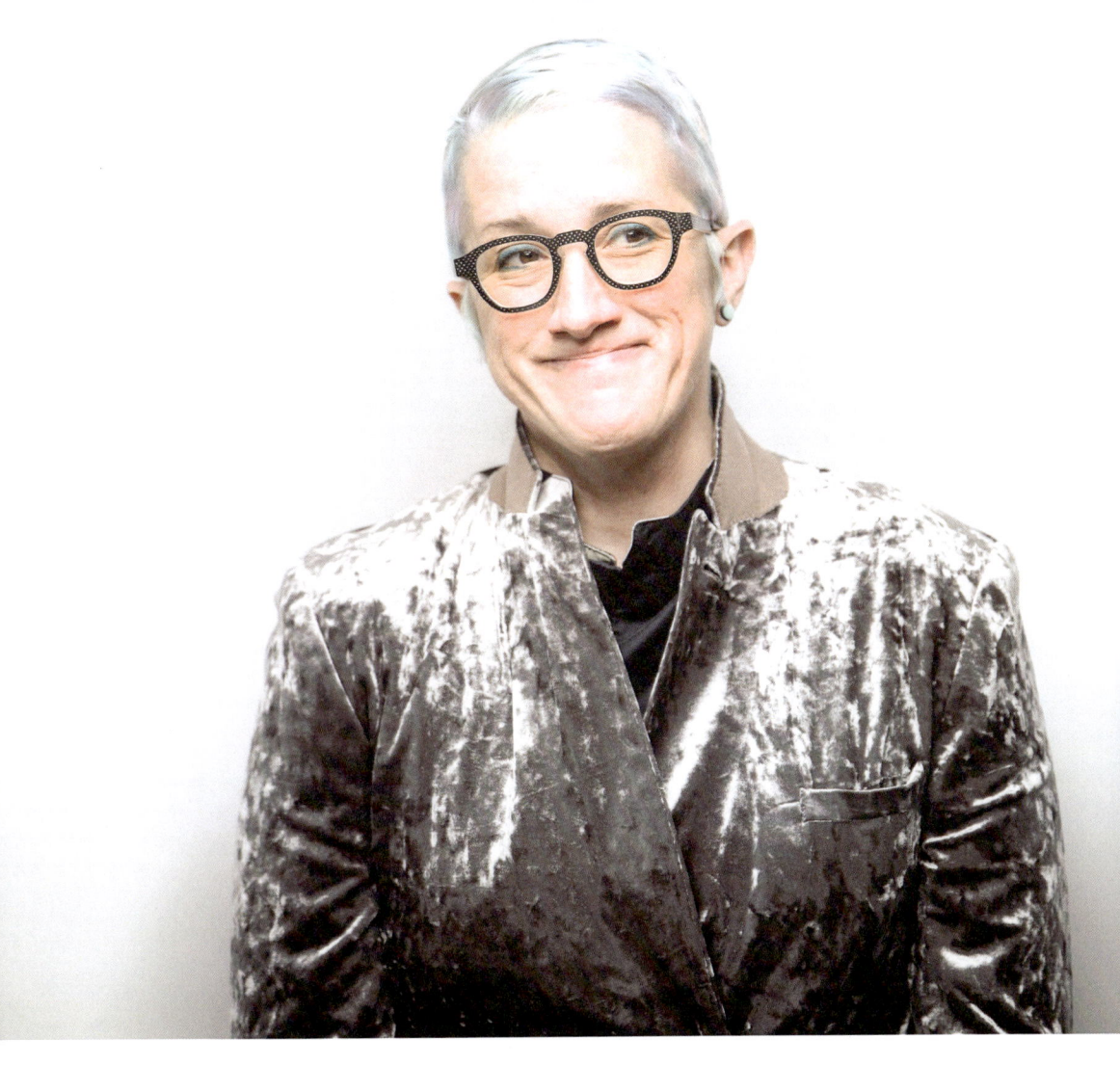

experienced professionals can guide and support families as they navigate their new reality with an individual diagnosed with autism.

Clinical Decision Support Technology is state-of-the-art in health care, but new to autism services and ABA therapy. Because the growth of this field has increased at a far greater pace than that of other health care fields, it's crucial that providers adopt technology to help them stay current on the latest data, trends, and best practices.

Ralston's passion for her work is evident in everything she does.

"I love seeing the lightbulb moments for clinicians when they realize how much easier our software makes their lives," she said. "I also enjoy working with such a talented and dedicated team."

Also, this isn't Ralston's first rodeo. She's a true cowgirl with a proven track record having founded two ABA clinics in two decades – the most recent of which (Verbal Behavior Consulting) was successfully acquired by the fourth-largest ABA organization in the United States in 2019.

AMBIGUITY AND ACCESS

LOUISVILLE NON-PROFIT CALLS FOR LEGISLATION TO CLARIFY HIV SELF-TESTING REGULATION IN KENTUCKY.

Caleb Bridgewater *he/him*

Inequity increases the likelihood of worse health outcomes and steals agency from us all.

Out-of-date restrictions on in-home HIV test kits have created inequity in access to these tests for Kentuckians that can't afford to buy them at the store or face stigma in their communities. The Social Practice Lab, along with researchers at Norton Healthcare, the University of Louisville, and the Pacific Institute of Research and Evaluation have recently highlighted how this outdated restriction affects organizations seeking to address health inequities in the Commonwealth. Here, we summarize their recent appeal from Director Michael Kopp.

The Social Practice Lab is a non-profit that "invests resources into communities in order to address and narrow the health equity gap."

The Social Practice Lab, among other organizations engaging in HIV prevention and service programs in Kentucky, has faced cease-and-desist letters when providing in-home HIV test kits in the past. Access to in-home HIV testing is an accepted strategy for informing and empowering individuals. In Kentucky, however, organizations looking to address the gap in access to in-home HIV test kits face regulatory confusion from the state.

Kentucky law KRS 367.175 prohibits "the sale, delivery, holding or offering for sale of any self-testing kits designed to tell persons their status concerning human immunodeficiency virus or acquired immunodeficiency syndrome or related disorders, and advertising of such kits" and is a Class C felony.

In-home self-test options provide agency and remove the stigma for individuals. The OraQuick In-home HIV Test is the only FDA-approved HIV self-test kit available in the United States.

These tests can already be purchased from retailers, including Walmart, Target, CVS, and Walgreens across Kentucky. However, smaller programs have received cease-and-desist letters

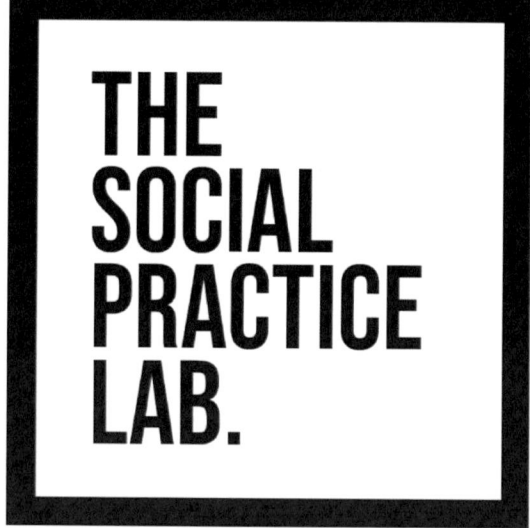

Image Courtesy of Michael Kopp, Social Practice Lab

www.ingramcontent.com/pod-product-compliance
Lightning Source LLC
Chambersburg PA
CBRC101144030426
42337CB00009B/72